Access to Health Services

Access to Health Services

Tulika Tripathi

GYAN

The Publication of this thesis was financially upheld by ICSSR and the responsibility of the facts stated, opinions expressed or conclusions reached are entirely that of the author and ICSSR accepts no responsibility for them.

ICSSR Consultant

Prof. B.K. Tewari, Head Political Science, Lucknow University, 302, Tirath Bakshi Apartments (New Hyderabad). Lucknow (U.P.)

ISBN : 978-81-212-1318-9

Price : ₹ 441

First Published, 2016

Published by

Gyan Publishing House
5, Ansari Road
Daryaganj, New Delhi-110002
Phones: 9811692060
E-mail: books@gyanbooks.com

Printed at: G. Print Process, Delhi.

Cataloging in Publication Data—DK
Courtesy: D.K. Agencies (P) Ltd. <docinfo@dkagencies.com>

Tripathi, Tulika *(Writer on public health)*, author.
Access to health services / Tulika Tripathi.
pages cm
Originally presented as the author's thesis (Ph. D.—Department of Economics, Banaras Hindu University) under the title: Public healthcare in Uttar Pradesh.
Includes bibliographical references.
ISBN 9788121213189

1. Public health—India—Uttar Pradesh. 2. Medical care—India—Uttar Pradesh. I. Title. II. Title: Health services.

RA530.U88T75 2016 DDC 362.109542 23

Access to
Health Services

Tulika Tripathi

GYAN

The Publication of this thesis was financially upheld by ICSSR and the responsibility of the facts stated, opinions expressed or conclusions reached are entirely that of the author and ICSSR accepts no responsibility for them.

ICSSR Consultant

Prof. B.K. Tewari, Head Political Science, Lucknow University, 302, Tirath Bakshi Apartments (New Hyderabad). Lucknow (U.P.)

ISBN : 978-81-212-1318-9

Price : ₹ 441

First Published, 2016

Published by

Gyan Publishing House
5, Ansari Road
Daryaganj, New Delhi-110002
Phones: 9811692060
E-mail: books@gyanbooks.com

Printed at: G. Print Process, Delhi.

Cataloging in Publication Data—DK
Courtesy: D.K. Agencies (P) Ltd. <docinfo@dkagencies.com>

Tripathi, Tulika *(Writer on public health)*, author.
Access to health services / Tulika Tripathi.
pages cm
Originally presented as the author's thesis (Ph. D.—Department of Economics, Banaras Hindu University) under the title: Public healthcare in Uttar Pradesh.
Includes bibliographical references.
ISBN 9788121213189

1. Public health—India—Uttar Pradesh. 2. Medical care—India—Uttar Pradesh. I. Title. II. Title: Health services.

RA530.U88T75 2016 DDC 362.109542 23

Contents

Acknowledgement

The dismal state of affairs in Uttar Pradesh and especially in eastern part of it makes any socially conscientious social scientist and one who happens to belong to this area, wonders how lofty goals of Millennium Development Goal can be achieved in this part of the world. Increasingly rising cost of treatment combined with poverty all around makes one despondent and hopeless. The state seems to have left it to the fate of its own. My interest on this theme arose when I happen to visit District Hospital, supposed to be the apex health provider in organisation of public health services, in my home town in eastern Uttar Pradesh. This motivation led me to my Ph.D thesis and subsequently to the present book. This book emanates from my earlier work on "Public Health Care in Uttar Pradesh" carried out as Ph.D thesis in the Department of Economics, Banaras Hindu University (BHU), Varanasi. I sincerely express my gratitude to all faculty members of the Department of Economics, Banaras Hindu University (BHU), Varanasi who have provided critical inputs in making of the initial draft of this book. I wish to put on record my utmost gratitude to my Ph.D supervisor, Prof Nripendra Kishore Mishra for painstakingly going through many drafts of the present book.

I am fortunate to have an opportunity to work in the Central University of Gujarat, Gandhi Nagar. It provided me the right kind of academic environment, incentive and infrastructure facility to complete this work which was pending for a long time. I am thankful to Prof S A Bari, Vice Chancellor, Central University of Gujarat and Prof N Rajaram, Dean, School of Social Sciences, Central University of Gujarat for providing necessary encouragement. This book has immensely profited from my discussion with my colleagues Dr Indira Dutta, Dr Jai Prakash Pradhan, Dr Vinod Sen, Dr Sarla Dasari and Dr Khasma Nidhi Adabar at Centre for Economics Studies and Planning and Dr Sudip Basu at Centre for Social Management.

I am especially thankful to Prof Amaresh Dubey, CSRD, SSS, JNU, New Delhi initially for his fruitful comments on my Ph.D thesis and later on encouraging me to look at nuisances of health data of NSS during my work with him. The present work also benefitted from comments of Prof P Kumar, Institute for Social and Economic Change, Bangalore. A brief stint at IGIDR under the mentorship of Dr Srijit Mishra was the beginning point of this book and Dr Mishra has always been a great source of critical inputs. I have been working on this project since last seven years and I have had discussion and comments from various eminent economists during this period on different parts of this book. It is difficult to name all of them. Yet, I shall be failing in my duty if I do not express my thanks to Prof Alakh Sharma, IHD, New Delhi. However, this book could see the day of light only by generous publishing grant from Indian Council of Social Science Research, New Delhi and I express my thanks to ICSSR for the same. Association with ICSSR was made more meaningful by the fact that Prof Pravin Jha reviewed this book proposal on behalf of ICSSR. I express my sincere thanks to Prof Pravin Jha. He has always been a great motivator for young researchers like me.

I am deeply indebted to Demographic Health Survey, Indian Institute of Population Science, Mumbai; Indira Gandhi Institute of Development Research, Mumbai; National Institute of Public Finance and Policy, New Delhi for the bulk of the data in this work. Special thanks to Dr Chandrashekhar of IIPS, who has provided me with relevant data and reports from time to time. The IGIDR committee members of visiting research scholars deserve a heartfelt thanks for the enlightened guidance they provided to me during my stint there.

Undertaking a project of writing a book, takes a heavy toll in personal space and one always need some people around to take care of that. My parents and my two brothers, Ashish and Rahul, filled that space during these years. My parents deserve special mention as they are ones who set me free to complete this work and always had good words to say during these years. I may have had disappointing times but they never had one. This support also came from my friends like, Hippu, Rekha, Garima, Deboleena, Punita, Reem, Manik, Binay and especially to Shashi. I am thankful to all of them. I also take this opportunity to express my thanks to B P Garg of Gyan Publishing House, Delhi and editorial staff of the same for making this work readable and presentable to larger audience.

Last, but not the least, I am deeply grateful to many others who has been directly or indirectly helpful during making of this book.

Tulika Tripathi

Preface

Uttar Pradesh (UP) is one such state which bears high population pressure along with very low social and economic development. It has the highest birth rate and the lowest life expectancy at birth among the major fifteen states of India. UP is performing poorly not only in demographic indicators but also in all indicators of development. It has the highest concentration of poor across the Indian states. Its per capita expenditure on health is amongst the lowest across states in India. Moreover in real terms it has stagnated over the last decades, which resulted into poor and inadequate public health infrastructure. Very high cost in private health sector and poor and inadequate health facilities by public providers has worked as deterrent for the poor and marginalised in getting the vital healthcare. Therefore, Uttar Pradesh is one such state which characterises all the features and pattern of inequality in its most glaring form and this is the reason for taking up UP as an area of study in the present work.

There are only limited studies focusing on UP and particularly all the more less on its health sector. Moreover these studies generally focused on state level aggregates and overlooked the inequality at the regional and individual level. UP is a very heterogeneous state and any aggregative analysis is fraught with the risk of over simplification. Therefore, a disaggregated analysis of UP is required, as it can give different policy implications within the state for the different region. Studies in health economics mainly look at health services at a very superficial level and none has seen utilisation of health services in relation to availability, affordability, acceptability and utilisation of health services. Moreover, most of these studies have focused on the in-patient utilisation of services. The present work is an attempt to fill this gap.

The access to healthcare services has been disaggregated into three components:

1. Availability of healthcare services.
2. Affordability of healthcare services.
3. Acceptability of healthcare services which has been in the present work seen as the utilisation of healthcare services.

The present work is based on the secondary data sources and therefore also have some limitations owing to the lack of data and inadequacies in the data set itself. Therefore, the objective of the study is to examine the role of public resources in determining the access to healthcare services that is the accessibility, affordability and acceptability and utilisation of healthcare services across different administrative regions of UP, namely, Eastern UP, Central UP, Bundelkhand and Western UP.

It is shown that there is an urgent need for revamping healthcare delivery mechanism in the state of Uttar Pradesh in general and Bundelkhand and eastern UP in particular. Moreover the government need to ensure better functioning of public health centres by ensuring availability of health personnel and equipments and drugs, rather than over-emphasising physical infrastructure. The state cannot leave health sector to market forces simply because health sector is characterised by the asymmetry of information, existence of profit enterprise and externalities. This provides sufficient rationale for the government to participate actively and significantly to safeguard the well being of the masses in general and of the poor and marginalised in particular.

Chapter 1

Introduction

Health is intrinsically and instrumentally important. Now it is well accepted that any development programme is incomplete if it fails to improve health standard of any country. Of course, all nation states embarking on path of development after Second World War, especially those adopting planned development, did emphasis importance of health and education, but none actually succeeded in ensuring universal healthcare. Providing universal healthcare to its population has been one of 'directive principles of state policy' in India too. But at least initial 50 years of independence have belied these hopes. A welfarist state committed by the constitution did nothing substantial in these fifty years. The period after 1990s witnessed a shift in paradigm with the introduction of neo-liberal economic policy. Roll back of state, cut back on non-plan expenditure and entry of private sector into public space became buzz words and consequently access to healthcare became either limited or costly for a majority of population of India. Of late, there seems to be a re-emphasis on health, but in a form different from earlier times. Now a bipolar structure is being created whereby private sector has come into health sector in a big way (in form of corporate hospitals) and state has renewed its intervention in an even bigger form like National Rural Health Mission. However, degree of access to health in India is still very limited and it is characterised by differential access for different socio-economic groups. Even this differential access is anchored in variation in geographical space. While for a sufficiently long period of time healthcare in India was automatically identified with public provisioning, now it has been clearly established, especially with recent growth of per capita income, that access to public healthcare is limited to lower income groups only. In fact, the way price of healthcare has gone up in recent times, lower income groups have only public healthcare to access. Therefore, it becomes all the more important to understand degree and determinants of inequality in access to public healthcare. Inequality in access to health combines demand for and supply of healthcare. Health care in general encompasses public, private, NGO and non- profit making firm's provisioning of healthcare services and health outcomes of the masses. However public healthcare in particular is the provisioning and financing of healthcare services by the central or the state government.

Health equity concerns not only with health seen in isolation, but it incorporates the larger issues of fairness and justice in social arrangements including economic allocations and paying appropriate attention to the role of human life and freedom from illness and premature death (Sen, 2002). Health inequality can be disaggregated into two parts one is process inequality (inequality in access to healthcare services) and the other is inequality in health outcomes. According to this there happens to be injustice if there is lack of opportunity to some individuals, like if one don't have opportunity to achieve good health due to inadequate social arrangements or/ and constrains put up by community/ public resources as opposed to some personal choice (Sen, 2002). This gives the clear distinction between health achievement and capability to achieve good health, where the later occupies the central territory in general and health equity in particular. As also concluded by Culyer and Wagstaff (1993), in their study that equity in healthcare should entail distributing care in such a way as to get as close as is feasible to an equal distribution of health. Now what is more important in the distribution of healthcare services is the consideration of horizontal equity i.e. equal treatment for equal medical need, irrespective of other characteristics such as income, race and place of residence (Donnell *et. al,* 2008).

Earlier the social and economic condition, that act as a setting factor which make people ill and in need of medical care, was thought to be the important determinant of health of the population and medical care was thought to act as a prolonger of survival and improve prognosis after disease (Wilkinson and Marmot, 2003). In this context the social and economic determinants of health outcomes, which is a stock concept are discussed a lot in academics and among researchers and policy makers. Nevertheless, the part of universal access to medical care i.e. processes generating equity/ inequity, is clearly one of the social determinants as it is not only important for treatment after diseases but it has important bearings on the diagnosis and prevention of diseases. This has been substantially overlooked by the researchers as well as policy makers. According to a WHO research, analysing data from 1952 to 1992, income growth is less important for improving health outcomes than the other factors such as access to health technology (Bloom & Canning, 2001).

Access to healthcare services on the one hand is determined by socio-economic differential and on the other hand by public resources. However, socio-economic differences also affect the access to the resources (Mukharjee & Karmeakar, 2008). Therefore, the question is whether presence of appropriate public resources reduces the socio-economic disparity in access to healthcare? If yes, then what are those favourable conditions? These questions have not been addressed by the researcher and academicians. There are studies which have partially touched these issues, like effect of place of residence, poverty, income inequality, employment level or racial profile on access to health (Pickett and Pearl, 2001; Wilkson *et. al.*, 1998). Studies like Wagstaff (2002, 2004) and Filmer and Pritchett (1999) do provide strong evidence of linking government health expenditure to health outcomes. Bokhari, Gai and Gottret (2007) also came up with similar conclusion in their study of under five mortality and maternal mortality as an example of an outcome of secondary care.

But very few studies have introduced policy variables and public resources which reflect the level and type of social and economic services and infrastructure offered in a community/ region

(Lynch, 2000; Eddy and Donnell, 2008). There is dearth of such studies for developing countries like India. There are a few studies documenting the precarious health situation vis-a-vis. the provision of public health facilities in India. But most of them focus on access and quality issues which deter people from utilising government health services. Some recent papers have also investigated the links between non-utilisation and administrative factor, such as absenteeism among the health staff in the rural areas, as well as the presence of alternative informal sources of medical care (Banerjee, Deaton and Duflo, 2004). But none have investigated the role of public resources in an area as a potential determinant of the individual's decision of access to healthcare services.

It is widely accepted that good provisioning of public health services are key to improving health outcomes in both the developed and developing worlds (Gupta *et al.*, 2010). For example, the provisioning of public health services by Japan reduced population's exposure to disease, helped raise labour force productivity and life expectancy, despite lack of rise in wages and consumption (Johansson & Mosk, 1987). There are certain communities, regions and segments of the population who are particularly disadvantaged in terms of access to public resources. Moreover, the uneven availability of such resources further adds to the widening of health disparity among individuals. Therefore the adequate arrangement of public resources can act as a modifying factor with respect to the association between health and socio-economic status as measured by income, type of employment, education, and racial profile. So, it is important to look at the interaction between available collective resources and capabilities in production of equal access to health services.

There are systematic variations in accessing healthcare between urban and rural areas as well between males and females in each sector. However, this socio-economic inequality is subject to the availability of health facility among various states. Motivated by this fact the present study seeks evidences from inter-regional variation in access to healthcare services in Uttar Pradesh and on that basis tries to delineate the relevant factors that results into higher access or in-access to healthcare services for certain groups in some regions. The present work is concerned with the public provisioning of health services and its consequences on access and health outcomes of different socio-economic groups in different regions of Uttar Pradesh, supposedly one of the most backward states of India. In exploring these questions of contribution of public resources to individual's capacity to access health services, this study utilises some basic statistics like average and proportion, burden of disease, analytical tool of Displaced Ideal to generate index of access to healthcare services and Sen's body of theoretical work on capabilities approach.

Access to Healthcare Services: Theoretical Framework

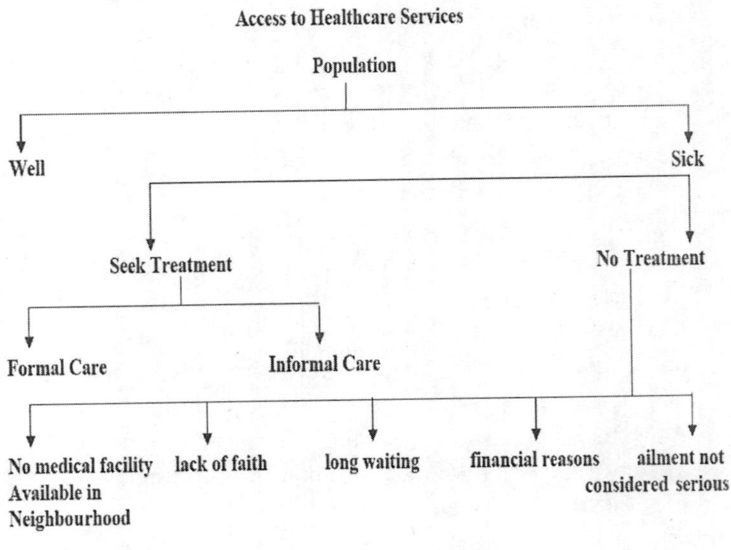

Access is the opportunity or freedom to use a health service and its utilisation. When an individual makes an explicit and informed decision to exercise his/her freedom to use healthcare, it is regarded as healthcare accessibility (Gilson & Schneider, 2007). The physical existence of healthcare facilities is necessary but not a sufficient condition for access. Apart from the physical existence, the people's ability to utilise those facilities and the quality of care available effectively determines the actual access. Moreover, the access to healthcare is also influenced by the attitude of the people to receive medical service, their knowledge about disease and the awareness of medical facilities (Simon, 2008). Therefore, access to healthcare can be defined as 'the potential and actual entry of a group of population into the health and healthcare delivery system (US Congress, 1988). In other words, it is 'the timely use of personal health services to achieve the best possible health outcomes including preventive care and ongoing care for health problems or emergencies (Berman, 2001). Thus, the access to health includes three factors; availability, affordability and acceptability.

Healthcare availability is supply side of healthcare, i.e., the condition of existing healthcare facilities. It refers to the physical existence of healthcare services at the right place and at the right time, which can only be ensured by the government. But only the existence of health infrastructure does not ensure its use by the individual, rather it largely depends on the financial access of services i.e. cost of healthcare and individual's ability to pay against the cost of healthcare. This plays major role in ensuring access to healthcare services. It is the capacity to buy healthcare services. Therefore, low cost of healthcare services makes it easily affordable to all, regardless of their money income. Besides these two factors another important factor is the acceptability of the healthcare services, i.e., the social and cultural distance between healthcare systems and their uses. It can be regarded as the willingness to buy healthcare services. Acceptability is a subjective thing which can be improved by literacy and awareness and knowledge about health programmes and their benefits to the individual.

Why Uttar Pradesh

UP is more than twice densely populated than the country as a whole, but has one of the lowest urbanisation; its per capita income was nearly half of the national average and about one third of Haryana and Punjab. UP has the fourth highest concentration of poverty among the states. In terms of literacy rates too UP stand at the bottom in comparison to other major fifteen states. It has lowest life expectancy (60) compared to the India average of 65 years. Similarly profiling the health sector all the indicators of health achievement like IMR, life expectancy, nutritional attainment, utilisation of health services and public health expenditure and health infrastructure it ranked at the bottom among major 15 states.

However in last several years, there has been progress on several health indicators such as the overall decline in childhood mortality, maternal mortality and incidence of preventable diseases. Still Uttar Pradesh is backward as compared to even some of the least developed countries (Chapter 3). Thus given the current trend, prospects of attaining the Millennium Development Goals (MDG) seem very difficult for UP (UPHDR, 2006).

Therefore the sheer population pressure and poor development status in Uttar Pradesh, leads to huge discrepancy in all the sectors in general and health in particular. The health outcomes across regions and districts with a few districts reflect a cluster of poor inputs and equally poor output – outcome indicators and therefore also reflecting the regional disparity in the state. The per capita expenditure on health is among the lowest across states and has stagnated in real terms over the last decade and a half. The poor delivery of health services through public health infrastructure is pushing people to the unregulated private sector for curative services (Srivastava, 2006,). The cost of accessing services, particularly hospitalisation services is prohibitive in relation to income thereby depriving the poor and the marginalised from getting the vital healthcare. Hence the small infrastructure and resources has to be shared among the great number of people, this obviously leads to all kind of inequality be it regional, social or economical. Thus Uttar Pradesh is one such state which characterises all the features and pattern of inequality in its most glaring form. Given such a gloomy situation of the state in general and health sector in particular there were very few studies on Uttar Pradesh. Some of the studies which are there mainly focused on the state level analysis that too in terms of general unequal distribution in the entire sectors i.e. education, health, income and employment etc. These studies have overlooked the inherent inequality at the regional or more micro level. However such kind of analysis may give a different kind of picture for socio-economic inequality in various regions and may leads to different kind of policy implication even within the state for the different regions.

Need for the Study

As mentioned above, the question of access to health and that too in context of public health has not received adequate attention in development literature. Of course, there are some studies for India, but this issue has not been examined either in context of interaction between demand and supply or at a much disaggregated sub national level. Moreover, its linkages with health expenditure are absolutely un-researched one. Uttar Pradesh is one state which has very critical role in terms of shaping overall development outcome of India, which in itself in a very poor shape. It is often said that India cannot develop by ignoring Uttar Pradesh. Least is known about health sector of UP. and absolutely nothing is known about pattern and determinants of access to public health in Uttar Pradesh, despite it being one of the focused states in NRHM. Therefore, a study which explores these questions is urgently needed. The present study attempts to fill this gap by carrying out this exercise for Uttar Pradesh at a more disaggregated level i.e. taking the four regions of the state.

Research Question

Therefore the present study is an attempt to explore the role of public resources in determining the access to healthcare services i.e. accessibility, affordability, utilisation and acceptability of healthcare services in various regions of Uttar Pradesh. Thus the explicit research questions answered in this piece of work are as follows-

1. What explains inequality in health? Is it regional variation or background characteristics of an individual?
2. Does better provisioning of public health services promotes equal and fair distribution of access to healthcare services and health outcomes?
3. How a compression of public expenditure on health affects access to healthcare and health outcomes?

4. Which section of population is the most affected by such compression?

Source of data- The data will be compiled from the following sources-

1. Financial Accounts of Uttar Pradesh and Kerala for Various Years.
2. National Sample Survey, 2004 - 60th round survey during January-June 2004 of morbidity and utilisation of health services. The findings will be based on published report as well as computation from unit record data.
3. NFHS – 3, the findings will be based on published report (Vol.- 2) as well as computation from unit record data.
4. DLHS – 3, the findings will be based on published report- Uttar Pradesh, as well as computation of unit record data.

Methodology

This study is based purely on secondary data source as named above. Some of the analytical tools used in the work are proportion and mean has been used to show the amount of availability of health facilities, morbidity pattern and health expenditure. To calculate burden of disease we have taken the ratio of average health expenditure to the average monthly per capita expenditure. Beside this range has been used to show the magnitude of inequality among various socio-economic groups.

Against this background the thesis is structured as follows-

It has been divided into six chapters of which the first three chapters set the background for the further analysis and conclusions drawn on that basis. The first chapter is Introduction in this chapter we initiated our discussion by signifying the role of health for an individual as well as society and nation as a whole. Further we have discussed the genesis of health inequality the issues concerning equity and inequality, the role of public provisioning in shaping and determining the equal and fair opportunity for healthcare services and health outcomes. Then we discussed why UP has been picked as the area for our research and then we put forth the dearth in the literature and thereby what we are intending to do in this piece of work that is our research question. The second chapter is the review of literature in which we have discussed the previous work in this area of study with a special motive to bring out the dearth in the literature and there we have discussed the gap in the literature at length regardless of it being answered in the thesis or not. Then the third chapter is basically about the scenario of Uttar Pradesh in general and specifically the health sector in reference to socio-economic and regional disparity. Particularly while doing so we have drawn some comparison from national average (India average) and from major 15 states also.

Subsequently from the fourth chapter we have started putting our answers of the research questions. It shows that there is a wide variation in public provisioning of healthcare services among the four regions of the state where in Western UP though having relatively less number of health centers but they are well equipped with health specialist, drugs and medical equipment. A good per centage of 24 hours functioning health centers also provides a good background for better access of health services and health outcomes in this region. Further pinning down the analysis reveals that however in terms of average health out of pocket expenditure in absolute terms is high in Western UP but the burden of disease is lower in this region. What is particularly important is our hypothesis about the public healthcare provisioning set the background for equal access to health services and health outcomes is stands true. As in Western UP the differential among socio-economic group is least in comparison to Bundelkhand and Eastern UP. We have also trying seen the acceptability and utilisation of public healthcare services among these regions and within socio-economic group; it shows some very interesting results for the sake of policy making that it is the larger number of poor and marginalised actually go to seek care from public health providers, therefore it necessitates the active role of government in better provision of healthcare services.

After that the fifth chapter tries to evaluate the results in above chapter in the light of public health expenditure. As the public healthcare expenditure is crucial for shaping the public provision of healthcare directly and indirectly the access to healthcare services and health outcomes. While doing so we have drawn comparision from the health sector of Kerala. It shows that over the period the neglecting policies for health sector, very low level and contracting health expenditure and more-over miss-matched expenditure has negative consequences for the health of the health sector. It has revealed a very important result that the public health expenditure although indirectly affecting is very crucial for the health of the poor and marginalised. As established in chapter four that it is marginalised and poor who are largely going to public health providers for their health needs and the rich and better off can seek care from the private health providers due to the high purchasing power and better negotiation power with the system. Finally the sixth chapter is conclusion which encapsulates the whole discussion and provides some policy implications and further study gap in the research. In Uttar Pradesh the level of health expenditure needs to be urgently revised. Seeing the high play of private providers specially given the scenario where the larger section of poor and marginalised are coming to them, it become all the more important that government come forward with policy relief (like universal coverage of insurance for the financing high cost of health services ensuring primary healthcare for all, better arrangement for preventive healthcare to check the spread of disease at the very outset and need based policies like policies focusing poor particularly in a state where still more than 70 per cent population reside in rural area) for poor and marginalised. Therefore in all likelihoods the government's active role is warranted in the health sector of Uttar Pradesh.

Work Cited

Banerjee, A, Deaton A and Duflo E (2004): "Wealth Health, and Health Services in Rural Rajasthan", *American Economic Review* 94, No. 2, pp. 326-330.

Berman, J (2001): "Turning Point Initiative", Colorado Department of Public *Health and Environment,* pp. 37, 40, 44.

Bokhari Farasat AS, Gai Y, Gottret P (2007): "Government Health Expenditures and Health Outcomes", *Journal of Health Economics*, 16: 257-273.

Bloom E. David, Associates P River and Fang K (2001): "Social technology and human health", Concept paper for the Human Development Report 2001, *Channeling technology for Human Development.*

Bose, A (2008): "India's Disturbing Health Card" *Journal of Health Economics,* Vol. XLII, No. 50, pp. 10-13.

Culyer AJ, Wagstaff A. (1993): "Equity and Equality in Health Care", *Journal of Health Economics*, 12: 431-457.

Donnell OO, Doorslaer V Eddy, Wagstaff A and Lindelow M (2008): *"Analysing Health Equity Using Household Survey Data: A Guide to Techniques and Their Implementation",* The World Bank Washington, DC.

Dorslaer V Eddy and Donnell O, (2008): "Measurement and Explanation of Inequalities in Health and Health Care in Low Income Settings", *UNU, WIDER*, Discussion Paper No. 04.

Filmer D, Pritchett L (1999): "The Impact of Public Spending on Health: Does Money Matter?" *Social Science and Medicine* 49, 1309-1323.

Gilson, Lucy and Schneider, Helen (2007): "Understanding Health Service Access: Concepts and Experience" in Stephen Matlin (Ed.) *Equitable Access: Research Challenge for Health in Developing Countries,* Global Forum Update on Research for Health Volume 4.

Government of Uttar Pradesh (2006): "Human Development Report of Uttar Pradesh", Government of Uttar Pradesh.

————(2006): "Uttar Pradesh Development Report – 2006", Government of Uttar Pradesh.

Gupta D Monica, B R Desikchari, Rajendra Shukla, T V somanathan, P Padmanaban and KK Datta (2010): "How Might India's Public Health Systems be Strengthened? Lessons from Tamil Nadu", *Economic and Political Weekly,* March 6, 2010, Vol. XLV No- 10.

Johansson, Sheila Ryan and Carl Mosk (1987): "Exposure, Resistance and Life Expectancy: Disease and Death During the Economic Development of Japan, 1900- 1960", *Population Studies,* 41(2): 207-35.

Martin MC (2008): "Individual and Collective Resources and Health in Morocco", *UNU- World Institute for Development Economic Research,* Research Paper No. 2008/21.

Mooij, J and Dev M (2002): "Social Sector Priorities: An Analysis of Budgets and Expenditures in India in the 1990s", *Development Policy Review* 22, No. 1, pp. 97-120.

Mukherjee AN, Karmakar K. (2008): "Untreated Morbidity and Demand for Healthcare in India: An Analysis of National Sample Survey Data", *Economic and Political Weekly*, November, 15.

Nathan, Mishra and Readdy, (2008): "An Alternative Approach to Measure HDI", *IGIDR, Mumbai,* Working Paper, 4.

Pickett, K. E. and M. Pearl (2001) 'Multilevel analyses of neighbourhood socioeconomic context and health outcomes: a critical review'. *Journal of Epidemiology and Community Health*, 55: 111-22.

Sen A (2002): "Why Health Equity", *Health Econ.* 11: 659-666.

Simon T.D (2008): "Health Care Accessibility in Kerala: An Analysis across Different Socio-Economic Groups" Paper accepted for Presentation at the Annual Conference on "*Equality, Inclusion and Human Development*" of the human development and capability association (HDCA), New Delhi, 10-13 September 2008.

Srivastava S Ravi (2006): "Health Security in Uttar Pradesh", in Prasad Sujata and Sathyamala C, *Securing Health For All: Dimensions and Challenges,* Institute for Human Development, New Delhi.

US Congress (1988): *The Quality of Medical Care,* Office of the Technology Assessment, Publication No. OTAH – 386, US Government Printing Office, Washington DC.

Wagstaff A (2002): "Intersectoral Synergies and the Health MDGs: Preliminary Cross-Country Findings, Corroboration and Policy Simulations.

————(2004): "The Millennium Development Goals for Health: Rising to the Challenges" World Bank Washington, DC.

Wilkinson R, Marmot M (Ed.) (2003): *"Social Determinants of Health",* IInd Edition, International Centre for Health and Society, WHO.

Chapter 2

Issues and Debate in Public Health Care

Recent development studies, in fact from early 1990s and after that, rely broadly on the development of human resources, which is defined as the process of enlarging peoples choice to lead a long and healthy life, to acquire knowledge and to be educated and to have access to resources needed for decent level of living. But of all these health is not only important but necessary constituent. The primary justification to focus on health is not only the fact that good health has other consequences, but that good health is a constitutive part of the quality of life that we can enjoy and is important in itself. Certain aspect of health sustain all other aspect of human flourishing because, without being alive, no other human functionings are possible, including agency and the ability to lead a life one has reason to value. It can be argued, therefore that public policy should focus on the ability to function and that health policy should aim to maintain and improve the ability of the masses of meeting health needs (Ruger 2004). This view values health intrinsically as well as instrumentally social good. It gives special moral importance to health capability; an individuals opportunity to achieve good health and thus to be free from escapable morbidity and preventable mortality (Ruger 2004). It has intergenerational impact too; often deprivation in health capability in one generation leads to further deprivation of health capabilities in the next generation, like the health of mother instantly affects child health. It has its instrumental role also as improvement in individuals level of income (due to lower expenditure on health, higher earnings due to better work opportunities and longer life-expectancy) raises individuals capacity to acquire higher education, increases families productive opportunities and greatly improves the psychological wellbeing of both the individual and the family. The benefits of good health will be even higher for the absolute poor, as they may transform the vicious circle of poverty into a virtuous circle with better nutrition, lower risks of unemployment, better housing, better use of training opportunities, higher productivity and better control over their life situation and that of their family.

Besides the benefit of good health to an individual it has importance for the society and nation as whole. It is important for acquisition of human capital and economic growth. Ill health means irrecoverable losses in production; a less well trained labour force as education and training opportunities are missed by those who are sick, larger health budgets, lower productivity in general, a less competitive economy, lower profitability of enterprises, higher labour force turnover and disruption in the national budget. Conversely, improvements in health will bring substantial benefits to the economy. Therefore it gives moral as well as profit value to have good health for all regardless of its creed, class, and any other differences.

I. Genesis of Health Inequality and Issues of Equity in Health

However there are many ways in which people suffer from preventable or curable health problem of any kind like medical neglect, general economic poverty, lack of social arrangement for healthcare and societal discrimination resulting into 'many faces of inequality in health due to the multiplicity of deprivation (Sen, 2004). Moreover individuals capabilities and functionings are not only determined by individual characteristics but also by social norms, that can impede ones optimal functionings and result into the inequality. In terms of sources of origin inequality in health sector can be grouped into two categories. First is the individual differences emanating from differentials in educational attainment, occupation and income. (IIPS and Macro International 2007 and NSS 60th round 2004). Secondly, it is generated by societal norms of stratification in the form of caste, class and rural/ urban divide which poses substantial threat to members of these categories to enjoy a healthy life (Thorat, 2007).

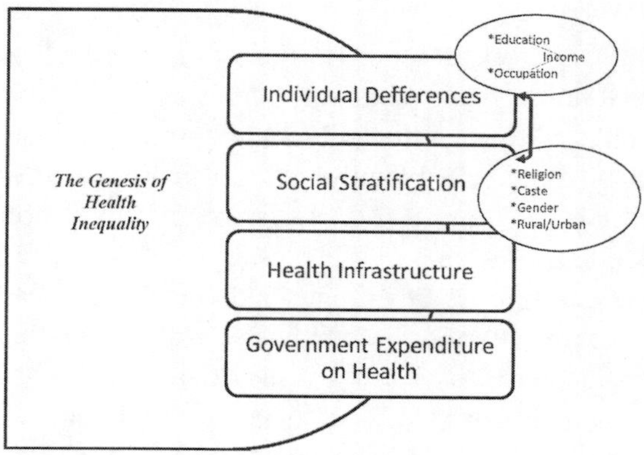

Fig 1: The Genesis of Health Inequality

Inequality in health sector is more like a vicious circle of poverty, once generated on one part of life, it is transmitted to other parts also like economically marginalised and uneducated fall into ill health and individuals with ill health remain economically and socially marginalised. The economic gains of the better off group helps them to further sharpen their skills which as a result enable them to corner out more of the benefits of economic opportunity in their favor. At the same time the social stratification in the society in terms of religion, caste, gender and rural/ urban divides leads to the lack of access to the various resources like education, good health facility and access to health specialist. Further, this stratification of the society leads to the high morbidity and mortality among these groups which is again closely linked with poverty and low educational (which generate lack of access) status of these groups. Moreover most importantly the health infrastructure also leads to the good/bad health outcomes, wherever health facility is unavailable or available at very high price it deprives a large number of the people to avail it and therefore compel them to suffer in bad health. Also, the high incidence of illiteracy, poverty and discrimination reduces their capacity to demand and utilise public health services.

II. Various Approaches of Health Economics

II a. Welfare Economic and Utilitarian Approaches

One of the leading frameworks for health ethics, policy and law is utilitarianism, which arguably serves as the standard framework for health policy analysis and was endorsed by the Panel on Cost-Effectiveness in Health and Medicine; they recommended Quality-Adjusted-Life-Years (QALYs) as the metric for ranking health interventions. Like most utility measure QALYs are based on the premise that utilities of different individuals and health conditions can compare on a single quantitative scale. It has been argued by health economists that treatment should be offered so as to maximise the total number of QALYs produced by the total population which is also referred to as health maximisation. However it has been accepted that age entered indirectly but it is obviously young people ceteris-paribus, who tend to produce more QALYs. If ageism involves inappropriate use of old age as criterion for exclusion, then an important ethical question is whether the indirect age relatedness of health maximisation is ageist (Anand 2004). Second when combined with facts about life expectancy differences between men and women, the fair innings appears to argue for prioritising the treatment of men over women (as women naturally gifted with longer life than men) which is very unappealing.

Other welfare economic techniques use different outcome metrics and include CEA and cost-benefit analysis (CBA) as well as CUA. CBA translates all benefits into monetary units through various techniques such as Cost of Illness (COI) studies, which value health outcomes by direct (medical and non-medical expenses) and indirect (lost productivity costs measures) costing methods. Willingness-to-Pay (WTP) and Willingness-to-Accept (WTA) methodologies use questionnaires to assess individuals willingness to pay for risk reduction or accept additional risk. CBA analysts also assess individuals preferences for changes in risk, based on their purchasing decisions and they ask people to assign a monetary value to various health states and associated risks, using Contingent Valuation (CV) surveys.

The application of welfare economic and utilitarian principles to health ethics, policy and law raises several concerns. First, accounting for only aggregate welfare without considering the distribution of benefits and burdens in society is problematic. CUA, CBA, and CEA tolerate significant inequalities in order to increase total or average social utility. Using utility measures to the exclusion of other measures also raises concerns. Sen (1985) has identified three main limitations of the utilitarian framework: (1) it omits freedom and focuses on achievements; (2) it omits certain achievements that are not reflected in the utility measure; and (3) it fails to measure accurately situations of persistent deprivation and adversity, in which people with significantly reduced functioning may not appear to be so deprived because they have adapted to their adverse environment.

II b. Communitarianism and Liberal Communitarianism:

Communitarian theories of justice argue that the provision of healthcare is an expression of community values and therefore, the justification for healthcare varies by community. Ezekiel Emanuel proposes a communitarian approach that incorporates aspects of libertarianism. He proposed a system in which the patients are given vouchers so they could choose among community health programs (CHPs) offering different levels of resources. He rejects cost-benefit, cost-utility, or cost-effectiveness methodologies because they bypass the need for collective reflection on values. His proposal has been criticized on impracticality and moral grounds because CHPs might be tempted to select benefit structures that favor some citizens over others.

II c. Egalitarian Theories: Equal Opportunity and Equal Welfare:

Egalitarian theories, a third framework, focus on the equal distribution of certain societal goods, one of which is healthcare. They do not support "equal sharing of all possible social benefits." Norman Daniels and colleagues have applied Rawlss theory of justice to healthcare and argue that healthcare is a right because it provides "equality of opportunity". Gerald Cohen has also drawn on Rawlss theory and expanded the Rawlsian view through an "equal opportunity for welfare or advantage" approach which supports rights for those disadvantaged by poor talents and skills as well as by disease or disability. Daniels counters that this interpretation places too little emphasis on choice or responsibility and raises problems for public policy including access to interventions that go beyond ameliorating disease. He supports the level playing field conception of equal opportunity, which requires efforts to eliminate or ameliorate social factors that limit opportunity over and above discrimination.

The Fair Equality of Opportunity (FEO) account does not discriminate among the different types of healthcare that society should provide its citizens under the "equality of opportunity" principle. Moreover, this theory does not consider the tradeoffs between healthcare and other social goods and adequately consider the costs of health insurance, goods, and services. Moreover, Daniels and others later extended the FEO approach to social determinants of health, claiming that health results largely from social conditions. Many have criticised this expansion, asserting, in particular, that the reduction of socio-economic inequalities might not necessarily diminish health inequalities. To solve rationing problems in the realm of healthcare, Daniels and his colleagues argue for "fair procedures" that solve rationing problems reasonably, although they have paid less attention to how individuals make rationing decisions and how to evaluate the outcomes such procedures generate.

The critiques of FEO tend to cluster around a few themes. First, FEO relies too heavily on statistical averages, which fluctuate with changes in the distribution of health and disease. Second, it does not include the alleviation of pain and suffering as a goal of healthcare. Third, it appears to exclude "non-productive" or "socially isolated" individuals. Fourth, it fails to clarify the concept of "fair equality of opportunity" and its link with healthcare. Fifth, indeterminacy and subjective valuation are implicit in the FEO account. A sixth area of criticism focuses on absence of guidance on weighing healthcare against other types of resources. A seventh points to insufficient consideration of "hard cases," such as patients with intractable and exorbitantly costly disabilities, who might receive unlimited medical services. Eighth, some critics argue that Daniels notion of adequate care is too vague to be effectively implemented. Finally, FEO is criticized as being too circuitous because the opportunity range is endogenous to the process of determining social investments in healthcare and other sectors.

II d. Libertarian and Market-Based Approaches:

Proponents of the fourth framework argue that a market mechanism is the ideal way to distribute healthcare. This approach generally stems from an overarching libertarian philosophy in which individual freedom and autonomy are the predominant societal values, and in which the governments role is to protect individual rights – especially property rights. This framework does not support a right to healthcare because efforts to guarantee such a right could infringe on individual liberties, by requiring people to pay taxes. Individuals are autonomous agents who may freely choose to purchase or forego health insurance or healthcare.

One of the main concerns of the libertarian perspective is that the conditions for efficient market allocation based on supply and demand do not exist in the healthcare or health-insurance markets. Although individuals have the right to make their own treatment decisions in many settings, they often defer to providers and insurance companies because of information asymmetry, uncertain health risks and limits on benefits. Moreover, consumers do not necessarily pay the full cost of healthcare or receive the full value of the goods and services they choose to purchase. Also, market failures – such as the public goods aspects of medical knowledge, the externality effects of communicable diseases, the failure to serve vulnerable populations, uncertainty, asymmetric information, moral hazard, adverse selection, and equity concerns – provide a rationale for public intervention in financing (and sometimes provision of) healthcare.

Another approach based on the free-market view is rationing through choice, which claims to accommodate diverse individual health and allocation preferences and thus respects autonomy. In this model, individuals ration healthcare at the micro-allocation level through ex ante choices among various health plans. The rationing-through-choice system, designed to use existing market mechanisms for healthcare delivery requires all individuals to contribute to a publicly funded healthcare system, which would fund health plans or provide vouchers for purchasing private or public plans. Plans that exceeded a certain government-allocated amount per capita would be more expensive to purchase.

II e. Deliberative Democratic Procedures:

In democratic approaches to allocating resources, citizens, as payers of insurance and consumers of healthcare, are involved in democratic deliberation and allocation decisions. One democratic decision-making model is the nformed democratic consensus model in which national legislature would set the overall budget for the plan, and the government would establish priorities and rationing protocols.

A number of criticisms of democratic procedures have emerged in the literature. Some argue, for example, that neither Daniels approach nor other theories of just processes are ever entirely culture-free, abstract or universal. Deliberative democratic decisions tend to be most difficult to implement, given the tendency to "rescue" suffering patients, even if their condition is not covered. Moreover, such deliberations would have to consider the costs and benefits of thousands of treatment options for thousands of diseases, a task too onerous to produce fair rationing policies. Another criticism is that majority preferences, no matter how well informed and fair, will sometimes eventuate in unjust outcomes. Therefore, a purely, or even primarily, procedural mechanism could return us to the same failures of justice that we have already encountered in healthcare.

While all of these approaches strive for a just distribution of health-care resources, one medical ethicist notes that "discordant positions, irresolution, and an exhausted uncertainty seem the only conclusive products of three decades of discussion on medical ethics." (Ruger 2006, p.112).

II f. Capability Approach:

Sens capability approach provided a possible solution to the limitations discussed above, in that it expands the evaluation space to consider. This theory is rooted in a particular view of good life and human flourishing. It states that quality of life a person enjoys is not merely a matter of what he/she achieves, but also of what options the person has (Ruta *et al.* 2007). In this perspective the capability approach takes a broader view because while accessing human development and quality of life, a focus on achieved functionings alone, like a focus on utility is incomplete, does not necessarily incorporate agency or freedom. In order to attend the foundational importance of freedom Sen introduces the concept of capabilities to take a holistic view for defining the quality of life. Capability refers to a persons freedom to promote or achieve valuable functionings. It represents the various combinations of functionings (i.e. doings and beings) that the person can achieve. Capability is thus the set of vectors of functionings, reflecting the persons freedom to lead one type of life or another, i.e., to choose from possible livings (Alkire 2002). Thus the notion of capability is essentially one of freedoms; the range of options a person has in deciding what kind of life to lead (Drez and Sen 1995). Part of this freedom relates to the availability of resources and how much these are deployed in a persons resource profile or capability set (Ruta *et. al.* 2007). Thus freedom entails both processes of action and decision and actual opportunities available to people, given their personal and social circumstances, in that both the process and opportunity aspects of freedom are essential to developing a just system.

There is much theoretical discussion of the application of the CA within the health economics literature and there are a few applications also (Anand 2004). The Capabilities approach valued health as inherent to the human condition and flourishing. Because without life itself, no other human functionings, including agency are possible (Ruger 2006). Thus it regards health as intrinsically and more highly solely instrumental social good. While discussing the economic growth and capability expansion Drez and Sen (1995) had seen health to be valuable to freedom in five distinct ways:

(1) ***Intrinsic importance-*** Being healthy are valuable achievements, in themselves and the opportunity to have it can be of direct importance to a persons effective freedom.

(2) ***Instrumental freedom-*** A persons health can help him/her to do many things e.g. they can be important for getting a job and more generally for making use of economic opportunities. The resulting expansion in incomes and economic means can in turn add to a persons freedom to achieve functioning that he/she values.

(3) ***Instrumental social roles-*** Good health in turn can help expand the facilities that the public enjoys and contribute to the better utilisation of the available services.

(4) ***Instrumental process roles-*** It broadens individuals horizons, and this can be particularly important for subalterns.

(5) ***Empowerment and distributive roles-*** It increases peoples ability to resist operation, to organise politically, and to get a faire deal. The redistributive effects can be important not only between different social groups or households, but also within the family. (Drez and Sen 1996, pp. 14-15).

The CA emphasises the multivariate nature of human well-being; there are many lists of human values that share this perspective. From this perspective it seems reasonable to suppose that core features of healthcare, such as mobility and pain, also have substantial implications for the quality of life. Indeed, it can be argued that health status is like income which is crude and imperfect measure. Just as some people can do more with fixed budget, so some people are able to overcome physical incapacity better than others. (Anand, 2004). Moreover, health status is not independent of well being in other areas of life. The practical significance of this point for human well being depends on the empirical relationship between health status and non- health aspects of life. Thus, QALY measure which looks at health status alone would be too narrow a measure on which to base the priorities. For example, two people might have same expected QALYs for the rest of their lives but quite different opportunities, because of their health status to seek and find paid employment. When it comes to deciding which of two individuals to treat, we might hold that their capacity to find work should not affect their rights to be offered treatment (Anand, 2004).

The CA suggests that wellbeing should be measured not according to what individual actually does but what the range of options and more importantly freedom he has to choose from. The main difference of CA is its evaluative space; it diverges from narrow utility space, which is concerned with the pleasure obtained from the consumption on goods and services and therefore to the maximisation of social welfare. Rather capability approach is based on what individuals are able to do and be, offering a realistic sense of their real freedom to pursue the lives they have reason to value (Ruger, 2006). Thus, the capability framework for evaluation is based on two distinctions, that between a persons agency goals and their own wellbeing, and that between achievement (functionings) and the freedom to achieve (capabilities).

The formulation of capability approach has two parts; freedom and doings and beings. In this perspective it is required that we do not simply evaluate the functionings but the real freedom or opportunities each person had available to choose and to achieve what they valued. Therefore, evaluation of equality must then take into account the freedom in opportunities as much as observed choices. This allows to takes into account the disadvantaged, marginalised and excluded. Thus Sen shifts the argument from resources and opportunities to achieved functionings and the freedom people have to formulate resources into the capabilities they valued and have reason to value. Capability approach views various states of well being which not only includes the achieved vector but looks at the whole process of the access and the conversion or utilisation the people make of the commodities (i.e. freedom to choose from various range of options).

From here two points of importance emerges for the evaluation of the wellbeing of an individual;

- Accessibility of the commodities and resources.
- Conversion of these resources into valued doings and beings (i.e. outcomes).

In health economics income is taken as a sole and major determinant of accessibility of health services and good health outcomes but the capabilities approach take it more than the income/ wealth only and tries to give a much careful description of the phenomenon and more suitable explanation of the causes. Sen recognises that the income has an enormous influence in what it can or cannot do but he underlines that instead of giving importance to commodities to live comfortably, we must put in first place the realistic life that people want to live i.e. the real life.

Sen explained it was more appropriate to evaluate the inequality through the space of capabilities than the space of utilities and primary goods. He stressed that we cannot translate automatically the possession of a good into well-being and he stressed that to possess a good is something different from the capability to benefit from the intrinsic characteristics of the good itself. This approach elaborated by Sen seemed to settle both the question i.e. the translation of all the available resources into the wellbeing of an individual mostly depends on the individual and the social characteristics. If we look at the achieved functionings we can observe the choice of the individual between a lot of possible vectors of functionings and they will reflect the liberty of choice made between different alternatives and the capability of doing it. The following figure illustrates this notion much clearly.

III. Measuring Access to Health

Healthcare Accessibility

To define access most of studies take it as the opportunity or freedom to use a health service and its timely utilisation. When an individual makes an explicit and informed decision to exercise his/

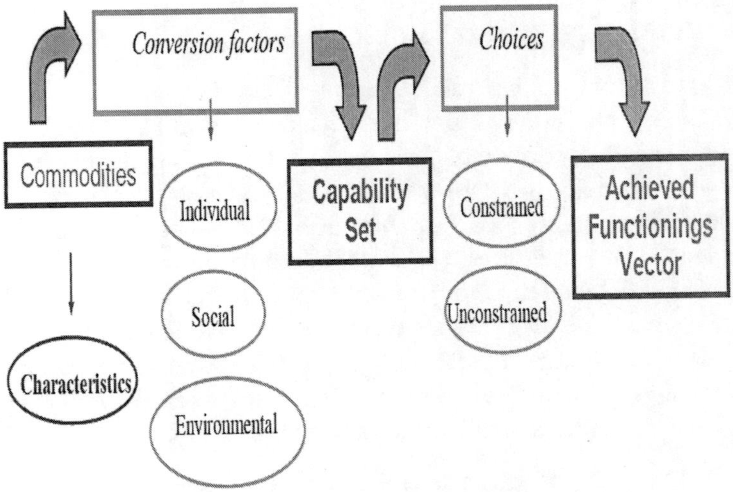

Fig. 2 : Accessibility and Conversion

her freedom to use healthcare it is regarded as healthcare accessibility (Gilson and Schneider, 2007). Most of them have taken indicators like ANC, institutional delivery and immunisation coverage to explain the access to healthcare across various socio-economic group or in terms of geographical coverage.

The physical existence of healthcare facilities is necessary but not a sufficient condition for access. Apart from the physical existence, the peoples ability to utilise those facilities and the quality of care available effectively determines the actual access. Further, the access to healthcare is influenced by the attitude of the people to receive medical service, their knowledge about disease and the awareness of medical facilities (Simon, 2008). Locational access, economic access and social access are broadly taken as a major component of access to health (Krishnan, 1999). However some of the studies reduced it to the quality of care and availability, including geographical accessibility, financial accessibility and acceptability of services (Peter *et al.*, 2008). There are studies which are of the view that among all the various factors that influence health, availability, accessibility and affordability of health services are more crucial and hence these need to be focused (Baru *et al.,* 2010).

Indeed one can have a clear picture of health system only when we can see utilisation pattern in relation to availability, affordability and acceptability. Therefore, access to healthcare is prerequisite for good health outcome (Baru *et al.*, 2010; Krishnan, 1999; Peter *et al.*, 2008; Simon, 2008). These variables are crucial in determining choice and utilisation of services. The access to healthcare can be defined as 'the potential and actual entry of a group of population into the health and healthcare delivery system (US Congress, 1988). In other words, it is the timely use of personal health services to achieve the best possible health outcomes including preventive care and ongoing care for health problems or emergencies (Berman, 2001).

Thus, the factors of accessibility can be grouped into three:

(1) Availability.

(2) Affordability.

(3) Acceptability and Utilisation.

Healthcare availability

Healthcare availability is the condition of existing healthcare facilities. Availability of healthcare is concerned with the ability of a population to obtain a specified set of healthcare services (Oliver & Mossials, 2004). Availability refers to the physical existence of healthcare services at the right place and at the right time.

Healthcare Affordability

Affordability refers to the financial access of services i.e. cost of healthcare and individuals ability to pay. It is capacity to buy a healthcare services.

Healthcare Acceptability and Utilisation of Health Services

Accessibility is the social and cultural distance between healthcare systems and their uses. It can be regarded as the willingness to buy healthcare services.

IV. Issues in Public Healthcare

In post-independence India what initially started as a programme for eradicating malaria and small pox, resulted in a huge infrastructure of public health in the 1950s and 1960s (Baru, 1999; Girish, 2009). During the 1960s and 1970s primary level health services grew, largely due to the pumping of funds for the vertical single disease control programmes and the family planning programmes. With too much emphasis on family planning, the PHCs lost orientation and curative health delivery services were neglected. Call it sluggishness or the sheer inability of the states to check these programmes, the downslide further escalated in the 1980s leading to a spurt in the private sector.

The mounting fiscal crisis and the stagnated expenditure in last two decades in the country turned out to be the fatal given such a dismal condition (Narayana, 1983; Baru, 1999; Girish, 2009; Duggal, 1997; Duvvury, 1999). Thus, the major problem with the health sector is essentially a cumulative effect of the following: a series of unfavourable developments coupled with misguided perception of the appropriate use of health sector infrastructure as well as the inability of the state to confront with the problems emanating from several sources plus fiscal crisis. Needless to say, the 1991 economic reforms had already cleared the deck for the stated purpose. However, with the unfolding of health sector reforms, there has been a paradigm shift wherein the conceptualisation of healthcare has changed from a service to a commodity (for which everybody has to pay) (Girish, 2009). At the same time there has been effort to mobilising additional resources for the health sector and therefore the scheme of user charges has been introduced which further put a setback for the marginalised and poor who are already suffering due to contraction effect of public expenditure.

In the 90s due to non-communicable disease, effective demand for healthcare from the emerging middle class and inefficiencies of public health sector in providing health delivery coincided with a budget constraint. At that time it was prejudice among both government and the public that private health sector will overcome the prevailing inefficiencies of the public health sector e.g. high absenteeism, low quality in clinical care, low satisfaction levels from services and rampant corruption (Acharya and Ranson, 2005). It was thought that competition among healthcare providers will reduce the cost of healthcare. But private sector took advantage of its being a priority or necessity of each individual. Each family will go for healthcare at whatever cost may be. Out of pocket expenditure was Rs 760,939 million (2005) which accounted for 72 per cent of total health expenditure and one which surely put a severe blow to the budget of any of the poor and middle class family (NCHM, 2005). They prescribe unnecessary investigations, tests, consultations, and surgeries as well as overcharge. Due to the fact that surgeries generate bulk of revenue to the hospitals, many are prescribed for it without any consideration of patients wellbeing. A study reveals that 31 per cent of deliveries were by caesarean. All these have increased substantially, out of pocket spending on healthcare (Nandraj, 1997). Tremendous increase in healthcare costs is revealed by the fact that hospitalised Indians on an average spend 58 per cent of their total annual expenditure. Over 40 per cent of hospitalised Indians borrow heavily or sell assets to cover expenses (Hammer, Aiyar and Samji, 2007). In addition, drug prices have also gone up recently.

Thus, the increasing cost of healthcare has made many deprived of attaining healthcare because market only serves to those who have purchasing power. Thus, the hardest hits by lack of health coverage are poor, who don't have money to afford it. They have much higher levels of mortality, malnutrition and fertility than do the rich. A study by the World Bank based on NSS 52nd round calculated that the poor rich risk ratio is 2.5 for infant mortality, 2.8 for under five mortality, 1.7 for childhood underweight and 2 for total fertility rate. In addition the study also indicates that a higher per cent of the poor do not seek care even when ill; about 24 per cent of poorest does not seek care compared to nine per cent of the richest. If one looks at the total illness episode treated during the last 15 days the poorest 20 per cent obtained treatment three times less than the richest 20 per cent. For hospitalisation the differentials is six times. Further the World Bank study concludes that the main reason for not seeking care is cost, especially for the poor (Gupta and Trivedy, 2005). The privatisation of healthcare has made a classification among society in terms of high level of disease for poor and low level for the rich (Hammer, Aiyar, Samaji, 2007).

IV (a) Privatisation of Health Sector and Shrinking Public Health Expenditure

There was substantial investment in the social sector in the 1950s and 1960s, the first two decades after India independence. Following the initiation of economic reforms in 1991, it was envisaged that the gradual withdrawal of the federal government from public sector shall result into the reduction of spending in the social sector. However, allocation for centrally sponsored health programmes continued to increase, up from Rs 208.17 crore in 1992-93 to Rs 489.71 crore in 1996-97 (Girish, 2009). However, state governments accounts for 75 per cent of total public health expenditure and therefore, what matters is the financial health of the state than that of the centre. Most of the state governments suffered from acute fiscal deficit (Girish, 2009) so as the UP government also. While WHO advocates for spending five per cent of GDP on health in India it is less than one per cent. Even, share of public expenditure in total health expenditure is only 15 per cent in India. The investment in health sector has gone down over the years, adversely affecting healthcare of the poor and marginalised sections of the society (Duggal, 1997; Girish, 2009). With the present level of allocation by the state to the health sector not even one- fourth of the health needs of the people are met.

Medical care (hospitals and dispensaries) and control of communicable diseases are crucial areas of concern both in terms of what people demand as priority areas of healthcare as well as what existing socio-economic conditions demand. As with overall public health spending, both these programmes also show declining trends in fiscal allocations in the 1980s and 1990s. In fact, in the case of disease programmes, this decline is surprising because of the large foreign assistance for AIDS and blindness control. This then means that for other crucial diseases like tuberculosis, the States increasing disinterest in allocating resources for the health sector (family planning being an exception) is also reflected in investment expenditure; there has been a very large decline in capital expenditure during the 1990s. Further if take into account the growth rate of inflation we would get a large negative growth for the most recent years. It is observed that share of centre in health expenditure is continuously declining and even the centres assistance is largely in preventive programmes as private sector is absolutely disinterested in this area (Duggal, 1997).

The deceleration in real per capita revenue and capital expenditure on health since the mid-1980s and the decline in the share of the heath sector in total revenue expenditure in several states are bound to undermine the role of public health sector in the provision of health services. Therefore, the presence of the state in the health sector has gradually shrunk. As a result for non-hospitalised treatment, the presence of government as a service provider has shrunk from 26 per cent in 1986 to 22.3 per cent in 2003 and for urban areas, it has fallen to 19.14 per cent in 2003 from 28 per cent in 1986. For hospitalised treatment, the government sectors share has fallen from nearly 60 per cent in 1986 to 41.7 per cent in 2003.

These figures cannot be taken to mean that people prefer to use the services of the private sector so far as healthcare is concerned. Private sector costs are almost three times higher as compared to cost in the public sector; Rs 8738 for hospitalisation in the private sector as opposed to Rs 3410 in the public sector. So for anyone with limited resources, it can be safely presumed that the public sector would be the default choice. However, given that public facilities are so poorly equipped, people do not have much of a choice. The NSSO figures show that on an average out of total sick persons 82 per cent in rural areas and 89 per cent in urban areas receive treatment of one kind or another. This per centage has remained fairly stable over the past 30 years. What has changed is the reason for which the remaining ill people do not take treatment.

As the presence of the public sector in healthcare is declining, the numbers of those who are unable to afford it are increasing. The people those who either had no money or were unable to find a local medical facility were 18 per cent of all untreated morbidity in rural areas in 1986, this figure shot up to 40 per cent by 2004. Even in urban areas, the numbers of those with no money for medical treatment doubled from 10 per cent to 20 per cent in the same period (Meeta and Rajivlochan, 2010).

The decline in public investment on health and the absence of any form of social insurance and safety net have heightened insecurities. The unpredictability of illness requiring substantial amounts of money at a short notice is impoverishing an estimated 3.3 per cent of India's population every year. The poorest 10 per cent of the population rely on sales of their asset or on borrowings, generating inter generational consequences on the family's ability to access basic goods and affecting their longterm economic prospects (NHP, 2006).

IV (b) Disjunction between Expenditure and Present Need

The blueprint for the development of health services that was outlined by the Bhore committee, both for short-term and long-term, emphasised preventive services, focusing on rural areas and linking health with overall development (Rao Mohan, 1997). Despite this the state responsibility in India in health delivery has always had a pronounced focus on curative rather than preventive care (Mukhopadhyay, 1997; Duggal, 1997), owing to the fact that responsibility for healthcare belongs to state governments while the responsibility for disease prevention rest with the central government. Often centres neglects this issue, but the state government has to treat the same at whatever cost necessary. This overall adverse effect of not preventing disease on national economy does not appear to have been appreciated by the Government of India or the Planning commission (John, 2010). It always had a strong urban bias, even as primary healthcare in the country has still a long way to go in terms of quality and coverage, given the fact that vast majority of Indians still live in rural areas (Mukhopadhyay, 1997).

The central government always influenced states financing in health sector despite health being states matter. This has been possible because healthcare policy-making and planning is largely done at the level of central government and hence the states just followed it. This structure of planning reduces any initiative that a state government may want to take for reallocating resources in favour of peoples demands for healthcare. The result is that people do not get satisfactory services from the public system and hence get discouraged to use it (Duggal, 1997).

Another serious problem in public health spending is the large and increasing proportion of the expenditure on salaries. This explains in part the poor use of public health services because non-salary component like medicines, fuel, equipment etc. are inadequately funded. The NIPFP database shows that commodity purchases declined steadily from 29 per cent of total expenditure in 1978 to 22 per cent in 1988 as did capital expenditure from nine per cent to 7 per cent. It also reveals that real growth rate in salary expenditure during that period was 9.8 per cent and that of commodities was 5.3 per cent (Tulasidhar, 1992; *cited in* Duggal, 1997; Duggal, 2006). NCAER also found in district and municipal level study in four states that non- salary inputs ranged between five per cent and 21 per cent (World Bank, 1994, *cited in* Duggal, 1997). This declining share of non-salary spending will aggravate the inefficiencies within the system, further damaging the already poor reputation of public health services.

The major problem of health sector development in India, especially in the last two decades, has been that new programmes are begun and new facilities are started with Plan funds (and an increasing amount with foreign borrowings) but their future sustenance is not completely assured by additional non-plan allocations. Health being a state subject, its sustainability is dependent on allocations made by the state. The centre has major control of plan resources and the states want to grab as large as they can. Therefore, in the initial years of the plan scheme they are willing to provide matching grants, but when it is time to take charge of the programmes they shirk from their responsibilities. The programmes then continue to remain a part of the plan resources with the result that new investments get affected because these old plan commitments do not get transferred to non- plan budgets. Further states have a tendency to divert programme funds away from components they are earmarked for. This is largely due to the restricted role they play in policy-making and planning. This mismatch of centre-state priorities have proved very expensive as funds are wasted on inadequately provided task causing allocative inefficiencies and failure of the programme to fulfil its objectives completely (Duggal, 1997; Rao, 1997).

IV (c) Increasing Cost of Healthcare

The far poor access to public healthcare services it has also been pointed out as a reason for increasing cost of healthcare services and its impoverishing impact upon individuals. However, most analysis tends to focus on the cost of hospitalisation as a major contributor to indebtedness. A nationally representative sample survey indicated that an additional 37 million Indians (3.7 per cent of total population) were impoverished in 1999 because of health shocks, increasing poverty head counts by 12 per cent (Meeta and Rajivlochan, 2010). In consequence, households out-of-pocket (OOP) spending is not only alarmingly high, but rapidly rising. This has serious repercussions by the way of catastrophic payments by households (Wagstaff and Doorslaer, 2003; Xu *et al.*, 2005, Doorslaer *et al.*, 2006). Moreover the public healthcare facilities which used to offer services free of cost have been forcing patients to procure drugs and receive diagnostic services from private service providers. This has grave implications for the cost of care even in public health facilities, which is responsible for the narrowing of cost difference between public and private sector health facilities (Selvaraj and Karan, 2009). Garg and Karan (2005) and O. Donnel *et al* (2005) have shown that approximately 11 per cent of households in India paid for medical needs which was more than 10 per cent of their total expenditure during 1999-2000 findings and about 2.4 per cent of population were pushed below poverty levels due to huge payments made for hospitalisation. Similar kind of results have been obtained by other studies also showing a considerable proportion of people falling below poverty line due to the catastrophic healthcare expenditure for inpatient as well outpatient care (Garg and Karan 2009; Van Dorslaer *et al.* 2006, Berman *et al.* 2010).

The OOP payment has proved as a significant drain on the households total resources as measured in terms of total consumption expenditure. The OOP as a share of total household resources increased from over five per cent in 1993-94 to approximately seven per cent in 2004-05. Because of low per capita consumption expenditure in rural areas, the OOP share accounts for more than seven per cent of total household consumption expenditure in 2004- 05, reflecting a significant pressure on household living status. In fact, approximately 14 per cent of household in rural areas and 12 per cent of household in urban areas spend more than 10 per cent of their total consumption expenditure on healthcare (Selvaraj and Karan, 2009).

People living in rural areas suffer from a large number of additional handicaps, like, their distance from urban centres means that service providers are unwilling to serve them, poor and unreliable communication system mean that it becomes difficult for them to travel long distances easily, their average incomes are lesser, their information base is also limited and life in farm settings means routine exposure to toxic chemicals, which in turn, increases their health risk. All these factors combined with the complete lack of any social security net renders them extremely vulnerable to sudden health emergencies and/or any prolonged illness (Meeta and Rajivlochan, 2010).

The declining public share in healthcare provision has direct implications for those who pay for healthcare services. Latest estimates for the year 2004 shows that per episode, the burden of medical expenditure on households for outpatient care is Rs 295, while for hospitalisation care it is Rs 7,116. Per episode the medical expenditure for outpatient care is Rs 214 in government facilities and Rs 286 in private sector health facilities. For hospitalisation cases, private sector cost is more than Rs 9000 per episode as against less than Rs 4000 per episode in government sector (Selvaraj and Karan, 2009). In the wake of escalating healthcare cost, largely led by private sector providers, both the catastrophic and poverty impact on the households have been substantial and rising (Selvaraj and Karan, 2009).

Further the drugs are also the significant cost drivers. On the demand side, drugs and medicines increase a substantial portion of the out of the pocket (OOP) spending by household in India. Estimates of NSS for the year 1999-2000 suggest that about half of the total OOP expenditure is on drugs. In rural India share of drugs in the total OOP is estimated to account for nearly 83 per cent while in urban India it is 77 per cent along with a meagre 10 per cent budgetary support, both of central and state government. Analysis of price trends shows that drug price are out stripping the price of all commodities. An examination of price trends of 152 drugs (consisting of 360 formulations) during 1994-2004 reveals that antibiotic drugs witnessed a price rise ranging between 1 to 15 per cent annually. In the case of anti-malarial drugs the price rise is mixed. Further the drug retail margins are extremely high in the pharmaceuticals market. This become evident when one compares the market price vis-a-vis the people procurement price of drugs (NCHM, 2005).

IV (d) Introduction of User Charges and Health Insurance

This strategy has been adopted to cope with the rising cost of healthcare and to serve ever growing populations with depleting resources. It serves three main functions namely, brought more autonomy in day to day functioning of hospitals, results into improved infrastructure and maintenance of establishment and hospitals are able to render services all through the year (Girish, 2009).

However, the experiences of both developed and developing countries have shown that introduction of user fees leads to further marginalisation of the poor (Creese, 1990). Sharif and Mondal (2009) have presented a comparative study of the impact of user fees in eight states. They come up with very noteworthy conclusions that user charges vary even district-wise in the studied states, except in Karnataka where the charges are uniform. Interestingly the charges are not only highest in U.P. but it is the only state where only of the entire user charges is retained at the source of collection and the rest goes to the state treasury.

The twin issue of equity and access of poor people to services are addressed through the mechanism of exempting BPL category patients but its implementation is constrained by several factors, like, all BPL families do not posses this particular identification card and there is lack of awareness among BPL card holders regarding their entitlement (Sharif and Mondal, 2009).

Illness is a leading cause of household financial crises in India. Visit any slum or village or any report or analytical paper will reveal the same story of the absence of an integrated public healthcare or universal social health insurance system, catastrophic payments as a major reason to plunge a sizeable section of even the well off to abysmal poverty levels (Krishna, 2004. Doorslaer *et al.* 2006. Garg and Karan, 2009). The health insurance schemes are generally targeted towards well off people in selected cities (Acharya, 2005). A study reveals this fact that only about 75 millions individuals may be covered by some form of health insurance in India, which is less than 10 per cent of the population. The rest of the population have to fall back on their personal source of funding healthcare expenditure. The higher growth of private health sector is catering to those who have the ability to pay (Gupta, 2005).

However, two government initiatives seek to provide safety nets to the poor by shifting the burden away from households. First the National Rural health Mission (NRHM) and National Urban Health Mission (NUHM) has sought to increase public spending to improve health infrastructure, strengthen human resources and decentralised delivery of healthcare services (Desai, 2009). Second, by introducing health insurance schemes to provide economic support to the poor and marginalised. The early step to alleviate such a burden is Universal Health Insurance Scheme launched in 2003. However, despite various modifications the scheme hardly evinced any response (Narayana, 2010). Then the government introduced in 2008 the Rashtriya Swasthya Bima Yojana (RSBY), a healthcare benefits package that covers up to Rs 30,000 for hospitalisation related expenses for families that hold below poverty line (BPL) cards. The goal is to extend coverage under RSBY to all workers in the unorganised sector, under the Unorganised Workers Social Security Act (Desai, 2009). It is two years since the RSBY has been launched and a limited evaluation is in order, however there are few studies revealing the unachieved agenda of RSBY (Narayana, 2010). At the beginning of the third year of RSBY, only in one-third of the total number of Indian districts (200) has been the enrolment of poor in insurance. In about 10 per cent of the districts (59) enrolment was in progress. About 125 of these districts belonged to just four states, namely, Uttar Pradesh (58), Maharashtra (27), Punjab (19) and Haryana (19). Together with Chhattisgarh, Gujarat, Bihar and Kerala these eight states account for over 85 per cent of enrolled districts. The rest of the 20 Indian states and Union Territories have hardly seen any movement towards enrolment of BPL families in RSBY. It is also evident that the proportion of poor families enrolled in the scheme varies between 39 per cent in Maharashtra and 81 per cent in Kerala. The states, such as UP, Bihar and Maharashtra, which have large number of poor households report low enrolment proportions indicating that the bulk of the poor is still not covered by the scheme (Narayana, 2010).

IV (e) Health Infrastructure and Access to Health Services; Shortage and Inadequate Distribution

In the health sector, the implication of ineffective state institutions meant, absence or near-absence of medico and para – medico personnel in remote areas, negligence on the part of health bureaucracy and medico personnel alike and lack of infrastructure including unavailability of Primary Health Centres, and Sub Health Centres in required numbers in the rural areas. This is not to deny that a massive expansion of rural health infrastructure had already been undertaken during the period of Sixth (1982-87) and Seventh Five Year Plan (1987-92). But the studies conducted during the second half of the seventh plan and also during the initial years of the Eighth Plan Period had revealed that PHCs were grossly underutilised largely due to inadequate staff, medicine, equipment, transport etc and also because the PHCs were mainly engaged in completing family planning targets (Duggal, Nandraj and Vadir, 1995). According to information derived from the Central Bureau of Health Intelligence (CBHI), Government of India, over the past 20 years, the ratio of the rural population to government doctors in rural areas has deteriorated, from being one doctor to 17,000 population for the country in 1986 to one doctor to 34,000 population in 2006 (CBHI, 1986-2006, *cited in* Meeta and Rajivlochan, 2010). Despite such abysmal numbers and the poor experience with community health volunteers since the 1970s, the government doesn't seem to plan any increase in the number of service providers in the public sector (Meeta and Rajivlochan, 2010; Duggal, 1997).

Two-thirds of private practitioners are located in urban areas when 70 per cent of the population resides in rural areas. Moreover, the public health sector too has an urban bias (Duggal, 1997 and 2006, Quadeer, 1999). As much as 80 per cent of public sector medical care services and consequently as much of the budget for medical care is for urban areas. The rural areas have PHCs which provide mostly preventive and promotive services, but not medical care which is the peoples main demand. Even four-fifths of the public hospitals and beds are located in urban areas (Duggal, 1997; Quadeer, 1999). Under the given circumstances the rural populace was left with no other option except turn to private practitioners, quite often trained in non- allopathic systems or flock to already crowded taluka/ block (sub- district) or district level hospitals. What aggravated the matter further was the progressive reduction in budgetary allocations in the health sector (Girish, 2009). The primary healthcare network in the country, consisting of community health workers, village health workers, Anganwadi workers, primary health centres and sub-centres, auxiliary nurse midwives, male multipurpose workers and PHC doctors, has failed to cater to the health needs of the rural populace. Absence of accountability, inefficient planning and inadequate resources have rendered PHCs and sub-centres built across country in many ways non-functional often lacking in doctors and medicines (Mukhopadhyay, 1997).

IV f. New Initiatives: NRHM and NUHM

In order to strengthen the reach and impact of health delivery services, the Government of India launched an ambitious National Rural Health Mission in April 2005. Its stated objective is to provide accessible, affordable and accountable healthcare to rural population in the country. The key components of the mission are locating ASHA in each village, Health and Sanitation Committee at the level of Village Panchayat (VHSC) for preparing village health plan, invigorating rural hospitals for effective services (both curable and preventive), measurable and accountable to community, minimising inter-state and inter-district disparities and above all ensuring unmet public health needs by integrating curative health concerns with its imperatives, such as safe drinking water, nutrition and sanitation and hygiene (Girish, 2009).

The latest performance audit of the National Rural Health Mission shows that the shortage of service providers at different levels across the country continues to pose a challenge (EPW, 2010). Each of the sub-centres is supposed to have an auxiliary nurse midwife (ANM), a female and a male health worker. The PHC is supposed to have a medical officer and an Ayurveda, Yoga, Naturopathy, Unani, Siddha and Homeopathy (AYUSH) doctor on a contractual basis. However, as the NRHM audit points out, while contract workers have been engaged to fill vacancies and 6.16 lakh Accredited Social Health Activists (ASHAS) have been appointed, the shortfall of medical care providers needs effective attention. In the 15 states it surveyed, 11 per cent of the PHCs were functioning without an allopathic doctor, while in 28 states and union territories, an AYUSH doctor had never been appointed (EPW, 2010).

Therefore, the National Rural Health Mission (NRHM), a flagship scheme for rural healthcare of the Government of India, continues to depend heavily on voluntary workers, whose main job seems to be to concentrate on preventive healthcare and on assisting people to reach the healthcare facilities at the Primary Health Centre (PHC) and Community Health Centre (CHC) level. Generating demand for health services is a laudable idea, but it needs to be accompanied by some plans to meet the increased demand, of the later, unfortunately, there seems to be no sign. For that to happen, a different kind of healthcare policy based on the ground realities of rural India and on existing systems of governance is needed (Meeta and Rajivlochan, 2010).

The Eleventh Five Year Plan proposed to introduce the NUHM as a thrust area which is expected to fill the lacunae created after the implementation of the NRHM and take care of the unmet needs in fast urbanisation process. Thus, with NRHM it would form the Sarva Swasthya Abhiyan. In keeping with the regime of health sector reform (HSR), the three key elements that were included are provision of essential primary healthcare services, appropriate technology through public private partnership and health insurance for the urban poor (Dasgupta and Bisht, 2010). Although there is no study on evaluation of NUHM, still the range of participatory processes that marked formulation of the NRHM has been lacking for NUHM. Therefore, urban health needs serious academic debate and survey.

V. The Gap in the Literature

After having a rigorous survey of the literature the following areas have been identified where almost negligible work has been done so far. No study has visualised access to healthcare services incorporating all its component of availability, affordability and acceptability and utilisation of health service and linking them together. The present study attempts to fill this gap. The health sector of UP besides it dismal state has not been studied in depth so far. There are some studies at state level mainly dealing with inequality in health outcomes and access to health services in terms of catastrophic health expenditure and people falling below into poverty. There is absolutely no study looking at this issue at a more disaggregated level. In a heterogeneous state like Uttar Pradesh, this disaggregation at the level of region or district is urgently called for. In the present work an effort has been made to visualize socio-economic inequality at regional level and then to locate district level variation in utilisation of health services and disease burden. There are many expenditure analyses relating it with the increasing OOP, health sector reform, privatisation of health services and its adverse impact upon health outcomes but very few have attempted to link it with the pattern of access to health services. This study does so and while doing that it draws comparison from Kerala. Howeverthere are still various issue needing academic attention and vigorous research like evaluation of various ongoing schemes like NRHM, NUHM and RSBY, RKS, JSY, etc. Further very few studies have been made on health insurance and safety net for the poor and marginalised and most importantly its linkage with access to healthcare services is something which is entirely missing in health literature. But these are issue outside the ambit of the present study.

Work Cited

Alkire S (2002): *Valuing Freedoms Sen's Capability Approach and Poverty Reduction,* Oxford University Press, New Delhi.

Anand P (2004): Capabilities and Health, *www.capability.approach.com/pubs/539anand_capabilities_health_pdf./.*, accessed on 10- 2-2010.

Berman Peter, Ahuja Rajeev and Bhandari Laveesh (2010): "The Impoverishing Effect of Healthcare Payments in India: New Methodology and Findings", *Economic and Political Weekly,* April 17, 2010, Vol. XLV No. 16.

Bidani B and Ravallion M (1997): "Decomposing Social Indicators Using Distributional Data", *Journal of Econometrics,* 77: 125- 139.

Creese A (1990): "User Charges for Healthcare: A Review of Recent Experiences", WHO, SHS Paper No. 1, Geneva.

Dasgupta Rajib and Bisht Ramila (2010): "The Missing Mission in Health", *Economic and Political Weekly,* February 6, 2010, Vol. XLV No. 6.

Deolalikar AB (1995): "Government Health Spending in Indonesia: Impact on Children in Different Economic Groups" in Walle D & Nead K, *Public Spending and the Poor: Theory and Evidence,* Johns Hopkins University Press: Baltimore.

Desai Sapna (2009): "Keeping the Health in Health Insurance", *Economic and Political Weekly,* September 19, 2009, Vol. XLIV No. 38.

Donnell, O., Heivan Doorslaer, Ravi R, Aparna Smanathan, Charu C Garg, Piya Hanvoravongchai, Mohammed N Huq, Anup K Karan, Gabriel M Leung, Keithin and Chitpranee Vasavid (2005): "Explaining the Incidence of Catastrophic Expenditures on Healthcare: Comparative Evidence from Asia", EQUITAP working Paper-5, Erasmus University, Colombo, Rotterdam and IPS.

Drez and Sen (1995): *India : Economic Development and Social Opportunity,* Oxford University Press, New Delhi.

Dreze, Jean (2004): "Health Check-up", *The Hindu,* 12 March 2004.

Duggal Ravi (2001): "Health Sector Financing in the Context of Womens Health" in Mukhopadhyay Swapna, *Women's Health, Public and Community Action,* Manohar Publication, New Delhi.

Duggal Ravi (2006): "Utilisation of Health Care Services in India" Ed. Prasad Sujata and Sathyamala C, *Securing Health For All: Dimensions and Challenges,* Institute for Human Development, New Delhi.

Duvvury Nata (1999): "Gender Implications of New Economic Policies", in Rao Mohan, *Disinvesting in Health: The World Bank's Prescriptions for Health,* Sage Publication, New Delhi.

EPW (2010): "Doctors for Rural India: What of the Proposal to Create a Cadre of Doctors Exclusively for Rural India?" *Economic and Political Weekly*, February 20, 2010, Vol. XLV No. 8.

EPW (2010): "Doctors for Rural India", *Economic and Political Weekly*, February 20, 2010, Vol. XLV No. 8.

Garg Charu & Anup Karan (2009): "Reducing Out of Pocket Expenditures to Reduce Poverty: A Disaggregated analysis at Rural and Urban and state Level in India", *Health Policy and Planning*, 24: 116-28.

Girish K (2009): "Introduction: Health Sector Reforms in India: Issues, Experiences and Trends", in K Girish, *Health Sector Reforms in India,* Manohar, Centre De Sciences Humanities.

Global Forum for Health Research (2004): Health Research for Policy Action and Practice, http://www.who.int/alliance-hpsr/resources.

Gupta Amit Sen (2004): "Misplaced Initiatives in the Health Sector", *People's Democracy,* Vol. XXVIII, No. 52, December-26.

Gupta D Monica, B R Desikchari, Rajendra Shukla, T V Somanathan, P Padmanaban and KK Datta (2010): "How Might Indias Public Health Systems be Strengthened? Lessons from Tamil Nadu", *Economic and Political Weekly*, March 6, 2010, Vol. XLV No. 10.

Gupta Sanjeev, Verhoeven Marijn & Tiongson R Erwin (2002): "Public Spending on Health Care and the Poor", *Health Economics,* 12: 685- 696.

IIPS and Macro International (2007): National and Family Health Survey-3, 2005-06: India: vl1. Mumbai, IIPS.

Jalan B (2004): "Health and Wealth", *Biblio,* March- April 2004.

Johansson, Sheila Ryan and Carl Mosk (1987): "Exposure, Resistance and Life Expectancy: Disease and Death During the Economic Development of Japan, 1900- 1960", *Population Studies,* 41(2): 207-35.

John Jacob T (2010): "Is India Ready for an Overhaul in Healthcare?" *Economic and Political Weekly,* May 15, 2010, Vol. XLV No. 20.

Krishna A (2004): "Escaping Poverty and Becoming poor: Who Gains, Who Losses, and Why?" *World Development,* 32:121-36.

Krishnan TN (1999): "Access to Health and the Burden of Treatment in India: An Interstate Comparison", in Mohan Rao, *Disinvesting in Health: The World Bank's Prescription for Health*, Sage Publications, New Delhi, India.

Lorgelly PK, Lorimer K, Fenwick E, and Briggs AH (2008,a): Outcome Measurement in Economic Evaluations and the Role of the Capabilities Approach: A Review of the Literature, Section of Public Health Policy, University of Glasgow.

———(2008,b): The Capability Approach: Developing an Instrument for Evaluating Public Health Interventions, Section of Public Health Policy, University of Glasgow.

Mayer (2004): *The Intergenerational Impact of Health on Economic Growth,* Global Forum for Health Research, Forum 8.

Meeta and Rajivlochan (2010): "Inequalities in Health, agrarian Distress and a Policy of Avoidance" *Economic and Political Weekly,* October 23, 2010, Vol. XLV, No. 43.

Mukhopadhyay Swapna (1997): "Introduction", in Mukhopadhyay Swapna, *Women's Health, Public and Community Action,* Manohar Publication, New Delhi.

Narayana D (2010): "Review of the Rashtriya Swasthya Bima Yojana", *Economic and Political Weekly,* July 17, 2010, Vol. XLV No. 29.

Prabhu Seeta K (1999): "Structural Adjustment and the Health Sector in India", in Mohan Rao *Disinvesting in Health: The World Bank's Prescription for Health,* Sage Publication, New Delhi.

Quadeer Imrana (1999): "The World Development Report 1993: The Brave New World of Primary Health Care", in Mohan Rao, *Disinvesting in Health: The World Bank's Prescription for Health*, Sage Publication, New Delhi.

Rao Mohan (1997): "Indias Augean Stables: The Unfinished Health Agenda" in Mukhopadhyay Swapna, *Women's Health, Public and Community Action,* Manohar Publication, New Delhi.

Ruger (2006,a): "Health, Capability, and Justice: Toward a New Paradigm of Health Ethics", Policy and Law, *Cornell Journal of Law and Public Policy*, Vol. 15:2.

————(2006,b): "Toward a Theory of a Right to Health: Capability and Incomplete Theorized Agreements", *Yale Journal of Law and Humanities,* Vol. 18:273.

————(2007): "Rethinking Equal Access: Agency, Quality, and Norms", *Global Public Health,* January, 2(1): 78-96.

Ruger P Jenifer (2004): "Health and Social Justice", *Public Health,* Vol. 364,

Ruta D, Camfield L, Donaldson, C (2007): "Sen and the Art of Quality of Life Maintenance: Towards a General Theory of Quality of Life and its Causation", *The Journal of Socio - Economics,* 36, 397-423.

Selvaraj Sakthivel and Karan K Anup (2009): "Deepening Health Insecurity in India: Evidence From National Sample Surveys since 1980s" *Economic and Political Weekly,* October 3, 2009, Vol. XLIV No-40.

Sen A (1985): *Commodities and Capabilities,* New York, Elsevier.

Sen A (2004): "Many Faces of Gender Inequality in Rethinking Society in 21st Century: A Critical Readings in Sociology" in Michelle Webber & Kate Benzanson, Canadian Scholars' Press Inc, Toronto, Ontario.

Shariff Abusaleh and Mondal K Subrata (2009): "User Fee in Public Health Care Institutions" Ed. K Girish (2009): "Health Sector Reforms in India", *Manohar, Centre De Sciences Humanities.*

Simon (2008): Health Care Accessibility in Kerala: An Analysis Across Different Socio-Economic Groups, paper presented at the annual conference of Human Development and Capability Association, New Delhi.

Thorat S (2007): Economic Exclusion and Poverty: Indian Experience of Remedies Against Exclusion, Draft Prepared for Policy Forum, Agriculture and Rural Development for Reducing Poverty and Hunger in Asia: In Pursuit of Inclusive and Sustainable Growth, IFPRI.

Unni J (2009): "Gender Deferential in Education: Exploring the Capabilities Approach", *Economic and Political Weekly,* Vol. XLIV No. 9.

Van, Doorslaer E, O O Donnell & R P Rannan- Elaja (2006): "Effects of Payments for Healthcare on Poverty in 11 Countries in Asia: An Analysis of Household Survey Data", *The Lancet,* 368: 1357-64.

Wagstaff, A and E Van Doorslaer (2003): "Catastrophe and Impoverishment in Paying for Healthcare: With Application to Vietnam 1993- 98", *Health Economics,* 12 (11): 921-34.

World Bank (2001): Engendering Development- through Gender Equality in Rights, Resources, and Voice. A Policy Research Report. New York: Oxford University Press. Cited in (IIPS & Macro International, 2007, *National and Family Health Survey-3, 2005-06: India:* vl,1. Mumbai, IIPS).

World Bank (1995): "Public Expenditure Management for Sustained and Equitable growth", *World Bank Report* No. 14680- PH, Washington.

Xu K D Evans, G Carrian and A M Aguilar- Rivera (2005): "Designing Health Financing System to Reduce Catastrophic Health Expenditure" Number 2, Technical Brief for Policy Makers, *World Health Organisation, Department of Health System Financing.*

Chapter 3

Public Health Care in Uttar Pradesh

India ranks at 134 position in HDI (UNDP, 2009) largely because of its failure to address some key components of human development, like health and education. Apart from lower health outcomes in aggregate, it is characterised by high degree of inequality in these health outcomes across different socio-economic groups as well as across states. In other words, health outcomes are mediated by regional and inter-personal differences. Individual characteristics like caste, religion, gender and place of residence are located into a particular regional context where state policy has important role to play. That is why SC, ST and women have generally bad health outcomes as compared to other groups in different region. As for example, health outcomes of socio-economic group from Kerala are always expected to be better than any other state of India and it is all the more so when compared to state like Uttar Pradesh. Uttar Pradesh is one and probably the most important one also, of the BIMARU states of India which are supposed to drag down India in terms of human development.

The state of Uttar Pradesh extends to over 241 thousand sq. kms., covering around 7.3 per cent area of India, is the most populated with its share of 16.2 per cent of countries population and fourth largest state of the country. The state has a total population of 16.16 crore as per 2001 census. It is a sixth largest political entity in the world. The state is marked by low levels of urbanisation with three quarters of household living in rural areas and only one quarter of household resides in urban area. The level of urbanisation has also been lower than most other states. The numbers of urban centres with more than one lakh population have grown slowly over last thirty years. The growth of rural towns with population less than five thousand have grown more significantly and these centres have grown in larger numbers in the western part of the state.

Administratively the state is organised into 17 administrative divisions, 71 districts, 300 tehsils and 820 development blocks. It has 628 urban local bodies and 52 thousand village Panchayats covering 97,942 inhabited villages (GOI, 2008).

Geographically the state can be divided into three distinct physiographic regions, 1- the northern sub-mountainous region called Tarai, 2- the Gangetic plains, a highly fertile zones covering around two-thirds of the area of the state, 3- the Southern plateau. For purpose of planning the state is divided into four economic regions i.e. Western Region, Central Region, Eastern Region, and Bundelkhand (Southern Region).

Resource-wise UP is a rich region with its fertile soils, good climate, plenty of surface and ground water and diverse flora and fauna. The state thus holds highly favourable conditions for agricultural development. The State is, however, rich in surface and ground water resources. Over three-fourth of the sown area is irrigated mostly through tube-wells. Uttar Pradesh also has a fairly large canal network. It is also endowed with large forest resources as well as livestock resources. However, the forest area of Uttar Pradesh has declined from 52 lakh hectares to 16.9 lakh hectares, creating a serious environmental imbalance (GOI, 2007).

UP is inhabited by people of different ethnic groups, caste and religions. Almost 82 per cent households are Hindu and 17 per cent are Muslim and only one per cent belongs to other religions. Interestingly a highest proportion of Muslim resides in UP than in India as a whole i.e. 13 per cent. 25 per cent of household belongs to SC, one per cent belongs to the ST and 50 per cent belong to OBC. However, 42 per cent of states population is under age 15 and only five per cent is age 65 and over (NFHS-3, 2006).

The state ranks low in human development indicators; occupied 15th rank among 17 major states in 2001 with human development index value of 0.5442 against all-India average of 0.6281. However, in the year 2005, UP's rank slightly slipped to 16th position (just above Bihar only) but the absolute value of human development index increased to 0.5709 against all-India average of 0.6639 (GOI, 2007). It shows that Uttar Pradesh is lagging behind most of the states of India in terms of the major indicators of social development, especially health.

I. Growth Trajectory of Uttar Pradesh

During most of the planning period the growth rate of the economy has remained markedly below of that in the country as a whole. As a result, per capita income of UP which was Rs 259 in 1950-51 and which was very close to the national per capita income of Rs 267 is now almost half of that now i.e. Rs 4787 in 1993-94 is one of the lowest in the country except Orissa (Rs 4726) and Bihar (Rs 3620).

During the first twenty five years of economic planning UP's economic growth was extremely slow at around 2 to 2.5 per cent per annum, which was hardly above the population growth of the state. Growth rates in UP picked up in the fifth plan period and were equal to national growth rate in sixth and seventh plan period. However since the beginning of the nineties growth rate in UP declined significantly and touched the bottom around three per cent per annum during the eighth and ninth plan period. However, recent time has seen some revival of growth rates. Thus, growth rate of SDP which was only two per cent in the ninth plan (1997-02) jumped to 6.3 per cent per annum in the tenth plan (2002-07). Even then growth rates in UP remained significantly behind that of national average indicating that the state has not been able to benefit from the fruits of economic reform and higher growth at national level (GOI, 2008, p.13).

The most important reason for this slow growth rate in UP. is the low level of public and private investment. Per capita plan expenditure in the state was as low as Rs 25 in the first plan (1951-56) and Rs 32 in the second five year plan (GOI, 2008, p.15). Plan expenditure went up in the subsequent five year plans and stood at Rs 10903 in the eleventh five year plan (Figure 2a). The levels of per capita plan expenditure in UP have not only been low in absolute terms but have also fallen short of the average plan expenditure of all states. In fact the gap has even widened in the recent five year plans (Figure 2a). Plan investments as a ratio of GSDP declined sharply in the nineties due to the fiscal crisis faced by the state government. Thus, total plan expenditure which was around seven per cent of NSDP in the eighties came down to less than four per cent in the nineties. The same kind of pattern follows for public capital expenditure. Capital expenditure of UP is as low as sixt to seven per cent of total public expenditure and around 1.5 per cent of GSDP in the late nineties. However, there has been some improvements in last few years (GOI, 2008, p.16).

Being a poor state UP's capacity to generate substantial resources on its own for plan financing is limited. It is not able to attract a larger level of plan assistance from the centre. Central plan assistance to UP has been below average for all states throughout the plan period (Figure 2b). Moreover UP was not able to attract investments by central PSUs on any substantial scale. UP share of total investments in Central Governments undertakings was barely 4.8 per cent till 1980-81 (GOI, 2008).

On the whole a situation has emerged where UP is not considered as an attractive investment destination. The state being land locked did not find investors in major export industries. Moreover, the state does not have any mineral base and public investment in industrial sector had been lower than what it should have been. Therefore, it lagged behind in industrial development. The private sector investments in social sector and infrastructure, especially power and roads has not been encouraging. However, in the late nineties the state recognised the importance of private investment and thus opened – up its social sector like higher education and technical education for private investors. Though this phenomenon has some negative effects in the form of price hike of these public goods.

The structure of state income shows that the contribution of primary sector has declined to 34.5 per cent of the state income though the sector still sustain 73 per cent of the total work force. This shows the continued pressure of working population in the primary sector. On the other hand, shares of secondary and tertiary sectors, were lower in the state at 18.2 per cent and 47 per cent, respectively against the national average of 22.3 per cent and 55.7 per cent (2008, Planning Commission). It means that like national economy, Uttar Pradesh is also being tertiarised.

II. Regional Variation in Uttar Pradesh

Distinguishing feature of Uttar Pradesh's economy is its regional imbalances. Uttar Pradesh is divided into four regions: Western, Eastern, Central and Bundelkhand. The Western Uttar Pradesh is agriculturally prosperous, relatively industrialised and has seen greater degree of urbanisation. On the other hand, Eastern region is the poorest, characterised by low agricultural growth, lower number of industrial units, and lower gross value of industrial products. Central and Bundelkhand regions fall in the middle category (Table 1).

The low per capita income in the state conceals sharp differentials at the regional and the state level. Western region of the state is relatively more prosperous as compared with the other regions, while Eastern region is the poorest. Per capita NDDP of western region is about 70 per cent higher than that of Eastern region, while the difference is only between 10 – 15 per cent in case of the other regions (Figure 3a, Annexure-C). The income differentials are even sharper at the district level. Per capita Net District Domestic Product (NNDP) in 2004-05 ranged from a low of Rs 5,687 in Shrawasti district to Rs 34,709 in Gautam Budh Nagar district, i.e. a difference of nearly seven times. Only one district of the state, namely, Gautam Budh Nagar had per capita income higher than the national average (GOUP 2007, p.106).

Urbanisation levels are very low in both the regions reflecting their low level of development less than 12 per cent of population in Eastern UP and 22 per cent of population in Bundelkhand region lives in urban areas as compared with the figure of 28 per cent in the Western region. The economic structure shows low level of diversification in both the regions (Figure 3b, Annexure- C).

Table 1: Indicator-wise Hierarchy of Regions According to the Level of Development

Indicator	*Inter Regional Position*			
	Western	*Central*	*Bundelkhand*	*Eastern*
Population Density (per sq. km) (2001)	II (767)	III (658)	IV (280)	I (776)
Percentage of Urban Population to Total Population (2001)	I (28.3)	II (25.1)	III (22.5)	IV (11.8)
Literacy Percentage (2001)	III (57.36)	II (57.58)	I (59.30)	IV (54.27)
Per Capita Income in Rs at Current Prices- 2004-05	I (14260)	III (12554)	II (13136)	IV (8232)
Rural BPL Household (2002)	IV (25.84)	I (56.63)	II (43.48)	III (46.70)
Gross Value of Agricultural Product Per Ha. Of Gross Area Sown (Rs) at Current Prices (2004-05)	I (31772)	II (29423)	IV (18749)	III (21317)
Percentage of Industrial Sector to SDP at Current Prices (2004- 05)	I (14.93)	II (9.45)	IV (5.43)	III (8.72)
Composite Index of Development (Based on 36 Important Indicators)	I (117.28)	II (101.61)	III (95.48)	IV (85.09)

Source: Planning Atlas UP, 2006.

Agriculture in the two regions has remained at subsistence level. More than 90 per cent area is under food grains crops in both the regions. Productivity of all major crops is lower in both the regions as compared with the state average. While the potential of agricultural development is constrained by lack of irrigation and geographical factors in the Bundelkhand region, Eastern UP has favourable conditions for agricultural growth in terms of soil, climate and water resources (GOI, 2008, p. 7).

Both the regions Bundelkhand and Eastern UP are industrially extremely backward. There were only 2.7 working factories per lakh of population in East UP and 3.9 factories in Budelkhand in

2002- 03 as compared to the state average of 7.7 and national average of 12.7. Economic growth in both the regions is constrained by lack of infrastructure particularly in rural areas (GOI, 2008).

Considerable variation in poverty levels are observed across regions of the state. In 2004 – 05 poverty ratio was 25 per cent in the western region, while Eastern region and Bundelkhand had a poverty ratio of 41 per cent and 39.8 per cent respectively. In Central region the poverty ratio was 28.8 per cent. However, decline in poverty has been much sharper in Bundelkhand and Central region, though it was relatively slow in Eastern region (GOI, 2008). Similar variation can be seen in the pattern of incidence of poverty in the regions of rural UP (Figure – 3c, Annexure- C).

III. Health Outcomes of Uttar Pradesh vis-a-vis. Major 15 States of India

Uttar Pradesh is the fifth largest state of India with about one sixth of countries population, but one which lags behind in all development indicators. Uttar Pradesh is characterises by all the features and patterns of inequality in India in its most glaring form. Since a very large chunk of population has very small cake to share, the incidence of inequality is very strong here. Uttar Pradesh had occupied an important place in the polity and economy of the country in eighties. However, over the years around in nineties growth rates have sharply declined and UP has slipped down from its celebrated position (GOI, 2008, Singh, 2000). Present scenario of the state is very dismal in all the areas of socio-economic development. Almost all social indicators of the state show that the state stands on 13th or 14th position among the sixteen major States. Bihar and in some cases Orissa, are the only two states which lag behind UP in terms of social development indicators like medical facilities, teacher-pupil ratio in primary schools, birth rate, death rate, infant mortality rate, literacy, per capita income, electrification of villages, per capita power consumption etc. Uttar Pradesh is often seen as a case study of development in a region of India that currently lag behind other parts of the country in terms of a number of important aspects of well being and social progress (upgov.nic.in).

Among 15 major states UP is at the bottom in achievement indicator and at the top in deprivation indicators. (See Table 2). In 2003-04 UP ranked 14th among the major 15 states of India as far as, Per Capita SDP is concerned. Its per capita income was nearly half of the national average and about one Third of Haryana and Punjab. It has the sixth highest concentration of poverty among the states. Only Bihar, Chhattisgarh, Jharkhand, Madhya Pradesh and Orissa had a higher poverty ratio as compared to UP. According to the latest estimate of the Planning Commission based on NSS 61st round, 32.8 per cent of the population of the state was living below the poverty line in 2004-05 as compared to the figure of 27.5 per cent for the country on the basis of uniform recall period. Around 80 per cent of the poor in the state live in the rural areas. On the basis of the uniform recall period, poverty ratio declined by 8.1 percentage points in UP between 1993- 94 and 2004- 05. Despite the substantial decline in the poverty ratio the absolute number of poor has remained

Table 2

States	*Total Population*	*Birth Rate*	*Death Rate*	*MMR*	*Literacy Rate*	
					Total	*Female*
	2001	**2007**	**2007**	**2004-6**	**2001**	**2001**
Andhra Pradesh	76,210	18.7	7.4	154	61.11	51.17
Assam	26,656	24.3	8.6	480	64.28	56.03
Bihar	82,999	29.4	7.5	312	47.53	33.57
Gujarat	50,671	23	7.2	160	69.97	58.6
Haryana	21,145	23.4	6.6	186	68.59	56.31
Karnataka	52,851	19.9	7.3	213	67.04	57.45
Kerala	31,841	14.7	6.8	95	90.92	87.86
MP	60,348	28.5	8.7	335	64.11	50.28
Maharashtra	96,879	18.1	6.6	130	77.27	67.51
Orissa	36,805	21.5	9.2	303	63.61	50.97
Punjab	24,359	17.6	7	192	69.95	63.55
Rajasthan	56,507	27.9	6.8	388	61.03	44.34
Tamil Nadu	62,406	15.8	7.2	111	73.47	64.55
UP	166,198	29.5	8.5	240	57.36	42.98
West Bengal	80,176	17.9	6.3	141	69.22	60.22
India	1,028,610	23.1	7.4	254	65.38	54.16

Source: Registrar General of India, Census 2001 and SRS.

high in the state. Almost six million people in UP were living below the poverty line in 2004 – 05 constituting over one-fifth of the total poor in the country (GOI, 2008).

Similarly in terms of social indicators like IMR, life expectancy and literacy rates, UP ranked at the bottom among major 15 states (see Table 2, Figure 1a, 1b and 1d, Annexure- C). It has lowest life expectancy (60 years) compared to the India average of 65 years though the incidence of morbidity (105 per thousand) in UP is very low compared to Kerala (205 per thousands). However, there has been progress on several health indicators such as the overall decline in childhood mortality, maternal mortality and incidence of preventable diseases in last several years. Still, Uttar Pradesh is lagging behind as compared to national average.

III (a) Infant Mortality Rate

As mentioned earlier also Uttar Pradesh has very higher infant death rate of 70 in comparison to the national average of 55 and ranked 13th among major fifteen states of India (see Table 1 and Figure 1b). All indicators of early childhood mortality in UP. are not only higher than national average but neonatal mortality, postnatal mortality and infant mortality is more than double of national average, child mortality is more than five times of national average and under five mortality is more than three times of national average. In all indicators urban UP is better than rural UP (Table 3). Interestingly, probability of survival of Muslim child is always better than Hindu child. All mortality rates are always higher in rural area and Hindu religious group. A child of a SC mother has lower chance of survival than any other caste groups. Wealth appears to improve child survival chances across all mortality rates. Here the education of women plays a very substantial role as the child survival chances of an educated mother (of ten or more years of schooling) are very high as compared to an uneducated mother.

The IMR shows significant intra-state variations. During the 1990s, the Bundelkhand region showed the highest IMR. The female-male variance in IMR across regions also makes an interesting study.

In all the regions of the state the female IMR is higher. In the eastern, western, and the central regions the ratio is not only tilted in favour of the males but also the differential is very substantial (GOUP, 2007, p. 81).

Table 3: Early Childhood Mortality Rates by Residence NFHS - 3

	NN	*PNN*	*IMR*	*Child Mortality*	*U- 5 Mortality*
Urban	40.7	23.6	64.2	19.4	82.4
Rural	49.4	25.4	74.8	27.2	100
Total	47.6	25	72.7	25.6	96.4

Source: NFHS-3 2007.

III (b) Maternal Mortality and Poor Maternal Health Facilities

It is a sad commentary on the state of affairs that 38,000 women die every year in the state while delivering a child. Almost half the deaths occur at home and another 10 per cent to 15 per cent mothers die on way to the hospital. In 1997, there were an estimated 707 maternal deaths per 100,000 live births (SRS, 1998) in UP. This was almost eight times higher than the MMR of Kerala and 70 per cent higher than the national average (436). Recent estimates however, suggest that maternal mortality in UP has now come down to 240 in 2004-05 close to national average and far above 95 of Kerala (Figure 1e). It also needs to be added that for every maternal death, twenty mothers start living a life compromised by morbidity caused by pregnancy related complications (GOUP, 2007).

Over the years different national surveys like National Family Health Survey (NFHS) and Reproductive and Child Health Survey (RCHS) have suggested that there is very high incidence of "abortion complications", "pregnancy complications", "delivery complications" and "post delivery complications". Equally sad part of the truth is that a large number of households in the state do not seek treatment for reproductive morbidity. The pregnancy complications show a very even distribution across the state. Relatively, however, western and eastern regions record a higher incidence of pregnancy complications. Also, pregnancy complications are much higher than both the post delivery complication and delivery complication. Even post-delivery complications seem to outnumber the delivery complication all across the state (GOI, 2007). A major reason for high MMR in the state is the poor quality and low access of women to maternal health facilities. Though 67 per cent of the mothers received some antenatal care in the state (NFHS-3, 2007), only 26.3 per cent of mothers had at least three ante natal care visits (Table 4).

Table 4: Trends in Maternal Care Indicator 2005-06

Urban	*NFHS-3 (2005-06)*	*NFHS-2 (1998-99)*
Percentage who Received Antenatal Care	79.3	63.6
Percentage who had at Least 3 Antenatal Care Visits	40.9	36.1
Percentage who Received Antenatal Care within the first Trimester of Pregnancy	40	39.7
Percentage of Birth Delivered in a Health Facility	39.9	36.8
Percentage of Deliveries assisted by Health Personnel	50.5	51.6
Rural		
Percentage who Received Antenatal Care	64.2	29.2
Percentage who had at Least 3 Antenatal Care Visits	22.6	10.5
Percentage who Received Antenatal Care within the first Trimester of Pregnancy	22.1	12.3
Percentage of Birth Delivered in a Health Facility	17.5	11.1
Percentage of Deliveries assisted by Health Personnel	23.8	16.1
Total		
Percentage who Received Antenatal Care	67.3	34.7
Percentage who had at Least 3 Antenatal Care Visits	26.3	14.6
Percentage who Received Antenatal Care within the first Trimester of Pregnancy	25.7	16.7
Percentage of Birth Delivered in a Health Facility	22	15.2
Percentage of Deliveries assisted by Health Personnel	29.2	21.8

Source: NFHS- 2, 1998 and NFHS- 3, 2007.

In UP, only about half of the total pregnant women get ANC services. Only around 11 per cent of the eligible population get full antenatal care while the corresponding figure for Tamil Nadu was

75 per cent and for Kerala it was 85 per cent. In 1998 only 35 per cent of the mothers received any ante natal care (NFHS II). This jumped to 67 per cent in 2005 (NFHS III). In the urban areas, ante natal care rose from 63 per cent to 79 per cent, while in the rural areas, it jumped from 29 per cent to 64 per cent. 14.6 per cent of mothers had at least three ante natal care visits in 1997-98 (NFHS II) in 2005 this jumped to 26.3 per cent (IIPS 2007). 24.9 per cent of pregnant mothers received antenatal care from Doctors. 13.9 per cent from ANM/LHV; 6.0 per cent from TBAs, 8.5 per cent from others and 49.2 per cent mothers received no antenatal care (NFHS III (2005). It is, therefore, that Uttar Pradeshs health scenario is marked by a very high degree of reproductive morbidity and mortality (Figure 4a, Annexure-C).

III (c) Safe Delivery

The proportion of unsafe delivery is also extremely high in UP with only 22 per cent of births being institutional delivery (GOI, 2008). Trained personnel provide assistance to around one-fourth of the total deliveries in the state i.e. 29 per cent of the deliveries. Three fourths of deliveries take place in unhygienic conditions at home (GOI, 2007).

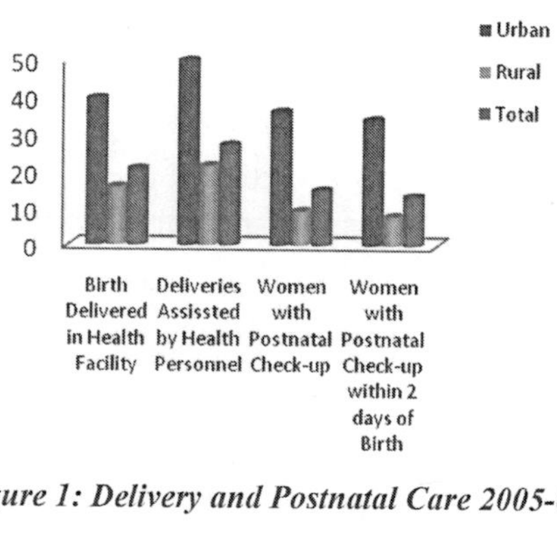

Figure 1: Delivery and Postnatal Care 2005-06.

There were only six districts of the state where more than 45 per cent of the women had safe delivery. Ghaziabad, Balia and Lucknow are the only three districts which record over 50 per cent safe deliveries in the state. Equally relevant is the fact that in different districts of UP only 03 to 42 per cent of the women were actually visited by ANMs and other health workers (GOI, 2007).

However Percentage of institutional deliveries increased from 11 per cent in 1992-93 to 15 per cent in 1998 and further to 22 per cent by 2005. In the urban areas it improved from 37 per cent to 40 per cent while in the rural areas it rose from 11 per cent to 18 per cent. The per centage of births that took place in medical institutions is about five times higher in urban areas than in rural areas. Inequity in utilisation of the institutional delivery services available is another very important issue. It becomes even more important given the fact that state is putting significant emphasis on institutional delivery. Only 8 per cent of the mothers who had institutional delivery came from the lowest quintile of the population, 11 per cent from the second lowest quintile while 46.6 per cent of the mothers came from the highest income quintile. Similar inequity is observed in terms of assistance received from health professional during delivery (Figure 1). Only 12.5 per cent of the deliveries in the lowest income quintile were supported by any health professional. 16.5 per cent of the mothers who received any health professionals support came from second lowest quintile while 58.9 per cent of the mothers who received assistance from any health professional in the state came from the highest income quintile (GOUP, 2007).

III (d) Immunisation

Vaccination against diseases has substantially impacted life expectancy as well as child and infant mortality across the world. In UP however a large number of children receive no vaccination at all. The change in vaccination coverage is a meager three per cent between 1997 and 2005 (Figure 4c, Annexure- C). The vaccination level in the rural areas is even more challenging than the state average. Intra state variations across different districts of the state are also very significant. The percentage of children aged 12 to 35 months who did not receive any vaccination ranges between 30 per cent to 54 per cent in different districts of the state. Interestingly, western region records lowest proportion of children who received complete immunisation. Even the proportion of children recording partial immunisation is found to be low in western UP. Eastern and central region present a much better scenario. It needs to be mentioned that while western region has a very high concentration of private providers, it lags behind in terms of public sector providers. As much of the immunisation is the result of public sector driven campaigns, eastern and other regions seem to have performed much better (GOUP, 2007).

Table 5

Vaccination	*BCG*	*Polio*	*Measles*	*All Basic Vaccination*	*No Vaccinations*
Urban	66.6	49.3	49.2	33	3.2
Rural	59.6	30.7	34.8	20.5	2.6
Total	61	34.4	37.7	23	2.7

Source: NFHS-3, 2007.

III (e) Malnutrition

It is alarming to note that UP has 52 per cent prevalence of under-nutrition, with every second child below three years of age suffering from chronic undernutrition. Surveys conducted in the state reveal that almost half the population in the 0-3 year age group suffers from various grades of malnutrition. Besides children, malnutrition in the form of Chronic Energy Deficiency is very high in women in the reproductive age group, aggravated by early marriage combined with early conception. On an average 80 per cent of pregnant women are anemic. Moreover, maternal malnutrition is often a major contributing cause of low birth weight babies (GOUP, 2007).

Besides the normal malnutrition challenge, UP also suffers from micronutrient deficiency. Micronutrient deficiencies are widespread in India. More than 75 per cent of preschool children and mothers suffer from iron deficiency anemia (IDA) and 57 per cent of pre-school children have sub-clinical Vitamin A deficiency (VAD). Iodine deficiency is endemic in 85 per cent of districts (GOUP, 2007).

Population density according to the 2001 census is 690 persons per sq. km. which is further rising. The decadal increase in population during the past two decades was close to 26 per cent. The annual growth rate of population stood at 2.33 during 1991 to 2001 much higher than the national average of 1.94 per cent. Of major states fertility in Uttar Pradesh is second only to fertility in Bihar. In UP. at current fertility levels a woman would have about three children during her life time compared with less than three children (2.7 children per women) in India as a whole. Fertility in rural areas is 4.1 children per women well above the urban areas of three children per women. Fertility rates are higher for women in disadvantaged groups (4.5 for SC and 3.8 for OBC) than their counterpart general women. The total fertility rates (4.3) for Muslims is quite higher than the fertility rates for Hindus i.e. 3.7.

Literacy rate in UP is (56.3 per cent) is very low when compared with States like Kerala (90.9 per cent), Goa (82.0 per cent), Himachal Pradesh (76.5 per cent) and Tamil Nadu (73.5 per cent). The ranking of Uttar Pradesh in terms of literacy is 31 in 2001 among a total of 35 States and UTs (GOI, 2007). Fifty four per cent of women and 21 per cent of men age 15 – 49 have never attended school. Only one- third of men have completed 10 or more years of education, but only 18 per cent of women have attained that level of education. Only 69 per cent of children age 6 – 17 years attends school in Uttar Pradesh, and this percentage is similar in urban and rural areas. 80 per cent of primary school age children (6-10 years) attend school (78 per cent in urban areas and 81 per cent in rural areas). School attendance drops to 73 per cent for children age 11 – 14 years and is only 40 per cent for children age 15 – 17 years.

Gender disparity in education is quite evident in the school age population in UP with 64 per cent of girls age 6 – 17 years attending school, compared with 74 per cent of boys in the same age group. However, the extent and direction of this gender disparity varies greatly by age and urban – rural residence. In urban areas, school attendance is higher for girls than for boys in the age groups 6 – 10 years (80 per cent of girls compared with 76 per cent of boys) and 11 – 14 years (78 per cent of girls compared with 76 per cent of boys). However, in the age group 15 – 17 years, 48 per cent of boys and only 43 per cent of girls in urban areas are attending school. By contrast in rural areas, girls in all age group are less likely than boys to be attending school, with the differential increasing significant, in rural areas, 84 per cent of boys compared with 78 per cent of girls in the age group 6-10 years are attending school and by age 15 – 17 years, only 49 per cent of boys and 28 per cent of girls are attending school (IIPS, 2007).

IV. Health Policy and Morbidity Challenge in Uttar Pradesh

Targets set by Government of Uttar Pradesh to achieve by 2012 in the following key indicators of health sector-

- Reduction of MMR to 350 per one lakh live births.
- Reduction of IMR to 40 per thousand live births.
- Under the RNTCP the target is to achieve a high cure rate of at least 85 per cent.
- 70 per cent detection of new sputum smear positive cases.
- Prevalence rate of one or less than one leprosy patient per 10,000 population.
- Under national blindness control programme reduce the prevalence rate from one per cent to 0.5 in UP by year 2012.
- Integrated control for vector borne diseases namely, Malaria, Kala-azar, Dengue, Japanese Encephalitis and Lymphatic Filariasis.
- To bring down total Goitre Rate (TGR) to less than 10 per cent. To ensure that more than 90 per cent household consume iodised salt.
- To ensure the availability of AYUSH system of medicine at an affordable cost, by ensuring that at each block PHCs, two medical officers, one of them being an AYUSH practitioner, are available all the time.
- Safe drinking water and sanitation facilities to more than 60 per cent of villages.
- Reduction of malnourished children by 50 per cent of present level.

Health scenario of Uttar Pradesh presents an exceedingly gloomy picture. As a matter of fact UP health indicators are not only below the national average but also lower than some of the poorer states. The incidence of blindness, tuberculosis, leprosy and maternal morbidity is also high. UP has the highest Disability Adjusted Life Years (DALYs) loss rate among all the Indian states (GOUP, 2008). And the most significant cause of these premature deaths is communicable diseases, malnutrition and prenatal conditions. The poor and the women seem to be at greatest disadvantage in sharing bad health.

Over the years, especially since independence there was a remarkable improvement in life expectancy at birth, birth and death rate and infant mortality rate, stated in the policy statement. Infrastructural improvement resulted in epidemiological shifts. Incidences of communicable diseases declined whereas sexual infections and emerging non-communicable diseases took its toll. It is the revelation that communicable diseases, lifestyle diseases and prenatal conditions are the major killers in Uttar Pradesh. In Uttar Pradesh on an average 105 persons per thousand has reported any kind of ailment in 60th NSS round which is far less than Kerala's reported morbidity of 205. Some of the major ailment (killer) and their detail are as follows -

IV (a) Leprosy Eradication Programme

In 1983 over 1,87,000 cases of leprosy were on record. Around the turn of the century, 50,000-60,000 new cases were being detected in Uttar Pradesh every year. However, by 2005 this number had come down to 27,582. The male-female ratio of the affected persons works out to approximately 2:1. The prevalence rate of leprosy was 52.7 per 10,000 in March 1983. It came down to 1.5 per 10,000 by November 2005. Uttar Pradesh is very close to the milestones of 1 per 10,000, which it has set for itself. Annual case detection rate was 2.4 against the milestone of 2.8 (GOI, 2007).

Leprosy is one of the major health problems in Uttar Pradesh, which falls in the range of high endemic states. The National Leprosy Control Programme (NLCP) was launched in the state in the year 1955 in two districts of the state. Later on, other districts were also covered. The Multi-Drug therapy was introduced in 1985, in Varanasi district. Since 1st April, 1995 all the districts of UP have been covered under MDT. With the introduction of MDT (Multi-Drug Therapy), the prevalence rate of leprosy has steadily declined.

IV (b) Malaria Eradication Programme

Malaria is a high incidence morbidity condition in Uttar Pradesh. The incidence of malaria shows a fluctuating trend (Fig. 4.5). On the whole, during 2000- 2005 malaria cases in Uttar Pradesh have fluctuated at around 85,000. The evidence suggests that over the years malaria cases don't seem to show any discernable decline, However, there has been a significant decline in death due to malaria. The RCH data also shows significant incidence of malaria in almost all the districts of the states. Maximum incidence is observed in the *tarai* belt i.e. eastern part of the state.

IV (c) Japanese Encephalitis Eradication Programme

Japanese Encephalitis (JE) is a much bigger and unique challenge in Uttar Pradesh. It is found that 60 per cent of total JE cases in the country are accounted for by Uttar Pradesh followed by the states like Assam, Karnataka and Bihar. In Uttar Pradesh the number of deaths due to Japanese encephalitis has shown a consistent rise from 35 deaths in 1994 to 476 deaths in 2006. The disease has emerged as a major killer particularly in the eastern region of the state. Around 32 districts emerge as worst affected by the disease.

IV (d) AIDS

Unlike the common perception, AIDS is very much a reality in Uttar Pradesh. There are at least 12 districts in the state which are regarded as high prevalence districts of HIV (see Map 4.2). Vulnerability profile of Uttar Pradesh for HIV / AIDS is very revealing. About half of the population is in the reproductive age group and literacy levels are extremely low. All this is accompanied by high incidence of poverty and high gender disparity. This substantially raises the vulnerability quotient of Uttar Pradesh as far as HIV / AIDS is concerned.

Efforts have been made by the state to meet the looming threat of HIV / AIDS. In order to ensure blood safety, 145 blood banks were established and strengthened in the state. Several voluntary counseling and testing centers (VCTC) have been established across the state. At least 83 centres have been opened in the District Hospitals, Medical Colleges and Government Organisations. These centres provide testing facility for symptomatic cases; provide counseling facility (Pre / Post test).

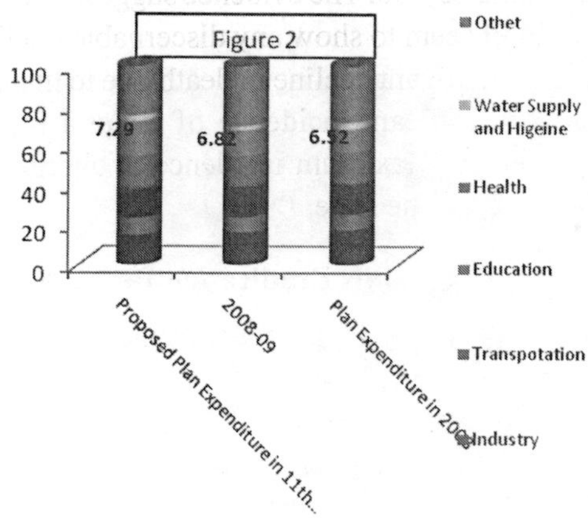

Figure 2

IV (e) Tuberculosis Eradication Programme

Tuberculosis is prevalent across all the districts of the state. But prevalence of the disease is much higher in Western and Central UP. While the detection rate is fairly poor, success in treating the cases is over 80 per cent. Sudden decline in detection rate during 2004 – 2005 is very noticeable. Understandably, there is a strong case for improving our detection system. Given the infectious nature of the disease, people remain in danger of being exposed to the disease.

V. Public Expenditure on Health in Uttar Pradesh

Main reason for the present dismal health scenario in the state can be attributed to the failure of public policy which did not pay adequate attention to health sector. This is reflected in the low allocations of the fund to the health sector in five year plans. In the first plan the share of the health sector in total plan outlay was as high as 8.50 per cent. During the next two plans the share dropped sharply to around four per cent. The downward trend continue in the later plans also. It was only during the tenth plan that an upswing was witnessed with the health sector being allocated four per cent in the total plan outlay. Per capita public expenditure on health in the state is extremely low barely around Rs 70 (GOUP, 2008). Whereas states like Kerala are expending almost double to the UP in per capita health expenditure.

The 10th Plan expenditure on health in UP was approximately Rs 1400 crore. During the 11th Plan this is proposed to 15000 Crore (including 2000 crore for Family Welfare Programme) of which 7500 crore or half will come from NRHM.

VI. Health Infrastructure – UP in Perspectives

Uttar Pradesh has a large public sector health infrastructure comprising one Super Specialty Institution (SGPGI),

Table 6- Health Infrastructure in UP.

Urban Areas		*Rural Areas*	
Type of Facility	*Number*	*Type of Facility*	*Number*
Super Specialty Institute	5*	CHCs	315
Medical Colleges	7- Government 2 - Central Gov.	BPHCs 3 - Private	823
District Male/ Female Hospitals	53	Additional PHCs + BPHCs	3640
Combined Hospitals	13	Rural PPCs	147
Urban FW Bureau	5	Sub Centers	20521
Urban FW Centers	61		
Health Posts	136		
District Level PPCs	63		

Source: Human Development Report Uttar Pradesh 2007.

seven government medical colleges and hospitals, 53 District Hospitals, 13 Combined Hospitals, 388 Community Health Centres, 823 block PHCs, 2817 Additional PHCs apart from 20521 Sub Centres (Table 6). Government has allowed private medical colleges to be set up in the state. Under this policy three medical colleges and hospitals have been opened. In addition, 4913 private hospitals / nursing homes have been established. There are a large number of registered and non-registered medical practitioners in the State, who are practicing in the state and they play an important role in providing medical service to the rural population.

However, the physical health infrastructure in the State is still much below the country average. Instance, the population covered by a Sub-centre in the State is 7080 and the average distance is 3.4 km., while the country average is 5109 and 1.3 km. It is estimated that 11 per cent of people in Uttar Pradesh are not able to access medical care due to locational reasons. Further, even when accessed, there is no guarantee of sustained care. Several other deterrents such as bad roads, unreliability of presence of the health provider, costs of transport and wages foregone, etc. make it cheaper for a villager to get treatment from the local quacks (GOUP, 2007). As the matter of fact in terms of physical and personnel shortfall in health infrastructure in comparison to India vis-a-vis, fifteen major states UP ranks at the top of the ladder (Table 7). The shortfall in CHCs is 75.23 in UP highest among Indian states whereas there are states which has surplus health infrastructure like Assam and Rajasthan. In terms of shortage in health personnel there were literature reporting the number of health centres running without specialist and health workers, in various states of India the shortfall of specialist is more than 75 per cent, while the shortfall of health workers is more than 50 per cent both for male and female, however shortage is quite alarming for specialist and male workers. It is clear that while the country has made some progress in improving the state of health of the people, but it is not uniform across the states.

In terms of physical and personnel shortfall in health infrastructure Uttar Pradesh is the worst state among major states of India (See Table 7). The shortfall in CHCs and sub-centres are 75.23 per cent and 22.1 per cent respectively. However, there are states which have surplus health infrastructure like Assam and Rajasthan. There is a severe shortage of health personnel also at all levels in Uttar Pradesh. Therefore every health functionary is under great pressure a large chunk of population which deteriorated the quality of care in public health sector. While the shortfall in specialist is more than 75 per cent, in case of health workers it is more than 50 per cent. On this basis it can be concluded that there were so many health centres running without specialist and even without health workers. Therefore the constrained supply side could be one of the probable reasons of inequality in states because it creates a mismatch in the demand (health needs) and supply of health facilities. This gap always affects weaker section more adversely than stronger section, as the latter will always be the first to grab the availability with their greater access to power and resources. Therefore, any shortfall in facilities is bound to lead to greater group inequality in health of the masses in the state. The situation is grave in terms of requirement of medical personnel *vis-a-vis* their availabilty, specially in case of doctors and specialists.

Table 7: Shortfall in Personnel and Physical Infrastructure in Health Sector of UP. vis-a-vis. India and States

	Personnel Shortfall				*Shortfall in Physical Infrastructure*			
	Speci-alist	*Male Worker*	*Female Worker*	*Average*	*Sub Centers*	*PHCs*	*CHCs*	*Average*
Anddra Pradesh	75.15	51.07	14.85	47.02	0	18.41	65.28	27.90
Assam	N/A	N/A	*	N/A	*	26.15	51.46	38.80
Bihar	62.86	86.08	15.66	54.87	40.44	33.79	83.92	52.72
Haryana	88.66	82.53	32.88	68.02	19.45	17.8	31.2	22.82
Kerala	73.13	16.25	6.15	31.85	0	0	45.69	15.23
Madhya Pradesh	53.43	25.74	13.95	31.04	15.07	31.20	35.25	27.17
Maharashtra	72.48	41.67	21.67	45.27	13.99	9.27	17.94	13.74
Orissa	N/A	42.77	6.08	24.43	18.62	*	20.89	19.75
Punjab	64.88	51.89	24.75	47.17	11.21	9.70	5.97	8.96
Rajasthan	55.49	76.18	*	65.83	*	*	13.14	13.14
Tamil Nadu	23.20	82.69	*	52.94	0	0	19.45	6.48
West Bengal	54.91	50.00	12.22	39.04	14.42	53.74	30.52	32.89
Uttar Pradesh	**73.25**	**72.07**	**9.43**	**51.58**	**22.10**	**16.63**	**75.23**	**37.99**
Rank of UP.	3	5	8	5	2	7	1	2
India	**58.44**	**56.71**	**12.62**	**42.59**	**13.13**	**18.57**	**38.90**	**23.54**

Source: Health Information of India,2005,*- Surplus, N/A- Data Not Available.

Although the State has a large presence of private health providers, it is mostly concentrated in the urban areas and is largely focusing on curative aspects. A survey of hospitals in the private sector, commissioned by the Government of UP, revealed that there are 2,592 private hospitals with total bed capacity of 47,269. There are 2,321 general hospitals that account for 92.4 per cent of beds in the private sector, 201 nursing homes with 2,506 beds that offer maternal and child health services exclusively, and 70 hospitals with 1,010 beds that offer specialty services (GOUP, 2007).

The problem of shortages is further compounded by the absenteeism of public sector health personnel in the State. A World Bank study captures the overall percentage of absenteeism and reasons for absence in different states of the country. 45 per cent of the doctors were found absent from duty in Uttar Pradesh. Interestingly, 14 per cent out of this 45 per cent were on leave; 9 per cent of them were absent without reason; and 22 per cent (i.e. almost half of total absenteeism) of the doctors were absent from the post because they were on official duty.

VII. Health Cost and Financing

The financial burden of illness in Uttar Pradesh is very high. While the policy is to provide free healthcare at the cutting edge the de facto situation is that care at PHCs is not free. Primary Health Centres are chronically short of medicines. Patients have to purchase medicines from outside. Cost of transportation, absence of doctors, wage earning losses, etc. also add up to the cost of healthcare. While the government charges nothing and is, therefore, short of resources, the people end up either paying from their life time savings or borrowing to receive inappropriate care from inappropriate provider. The expenses on medical care and hospitalisation continue to be a major reason for poverty in Uttar Pradesh (GOUP, 2007).

Average medical expenditure per hospitalisation case in rural UP in the public sector is estimated at Rs 7648 (Table 8). This is more than twice as much as the national average of Rs 3238. This does not include loss of household income. Even the cost in the private sector is found to be much higher in UP. than the national average. In the urban areas too the cost of healthcare in the public sector is much higher in UP than the national average. However, in the private sector it comes out to be lower than the national average.

Table 8: Average Medical Expenditure Per Hospitalisation Case in Rural and Urban UP

	Rural	*Urban*
Public	7648	5144
Private	9169	10351
Loss of Income	920	536

Source: NSS 60th round.

Healthcare in UP is primarily financed by private spending with out of pocket accounting for over 71 per cent of the total expenditure. Total non public sector spending accounting for 83 per cent of the

Table 9: Medical Expenditure (Rs) as Percentage to Total Expenditure per Person per 30 Days

Sector	*Item*	*59th Round Jan 03- Dec 03*	*55th Round July 99- June 2000*	*50th Round July 93- June 94*
Rural	Medical (institutional) PCE (Rs)	9.6	5.73	1.96
	Per cent	1.89	1.23	0.72
	Medical (non-institutional) PCE (Rs)	33.55	32.96	17.07
	Per cent	6.59	7.06	6.23
Urban	Medical (institutional) PCE (Rs)	10.62	7.2	2.35
	Per cent	1.35	1.04	0.6
	Medical (non-institutional) PCE (Rs)	39.74	35.31	16.65
	Per cent	5.06	5.11	4.28

Source: NSS Various Rounds.

spending and the government healthcare funding accounting for only 17 per cent of the total spend. National Health Accounts estimates indicate that the household sector spends Rs 17158 crore on health in UP whereas government spends only Rs 2650 crore. Table 9, gives the picture of monthly expenditure on health according to various rounds of NSS for rural and urban UP. In rural UP in 2003 non-institutional medical expenditure accounts for 6.6 per cent of the total expenditure while institutional medical expenditure accounts for 1.9 per cent of total expenditure. Non-institutional expenditure in rural UP compares unfavourably with such expenditure than the national average. In urban UP too the non-institutional expenditure is found to be significantly higher. In absolute sense the expenditure in UP is lower, however, in percentage terms it is found to be higher.

VIII. Utilisation of Health Services in UP

It is alarming to find that only around 10 per cent of the people seek outpatient care from public facilities in rural Uttar Pradesh. Against this at the national level the percentage of people seeking outpatient care from public facilities is 22 per cent in the rural areas. In the urban areas, only 13 per cent of the people seek outpatient care from public facilities against the national average of 19 per cent. The role of public facilities in patient care is somewhat better. In rural UP, 27 per cent of the people seek inpatient care from public sector against a national average of 42 per cent. In urban areas the state picture is very close to the national picture. Thirty one per cent of the people seek inpatient care from public sector facilities against the national average of 38 per cent. It need be noted, however, that the rural facilities like CHC and PHC have 30 beds and 6 beds respectively hardly ten per cent of this facility is utilised. Thus, there is much scope for improved inpatient care in public facilities if bed utilisation can be improved (GOUP, 2007, Figure 5a & 5b, Annexure- C).

IX. Department of Medical, Health and Family Welfare, Uttar Pradesh

It is playing a vital role in improving the health status and quality of living of the people of Uttar Pradesh. The department has been involved in service of mankind since its very inception in 1921. The Department initially provided its services under the name of "Provincial Subordinate Medical and Provincial Medical Services". In 1946, it was divided into "PMS - I and PMS - II Services and Provincial Health Services (PHS). In 1964, P.M.S- I and P.M.S- II were unified to form the Provincial Medical Services (PMS). On 26 June 1973 the PMS and PHS were unified to form the present "Provincial Medical and Health Services". This department is responsible for providing Medical, Health and Family Welfare related services to the densely populated state of Uttar Pradesh (16,60,52,859) spread over a vast area of 2,40,982 sq.km. With the objective of providing health services in Urban and Remote areas, the department provides three-tier medical services in the state of Uttar Pradesh. Under this, at the first level, Health Services are provided in urban areas. Health services at the second and third level are provided in rural areas.

Level 1

First level Health Services are provided in Urban areas through District Male and Female or Combined Hospitals and are at district level. These hospitals are generally 100 – 500 bedded Hospitals, where various medical facilities are provided. At present there are 80 District Level Hospitals, 6 Combined Hospitals and 63 Female Hospitals are available.

Level 2

At this level health services are provided through Community Health Centres established at the Tehsil and Block Level. Presently the standard for setting up the CHC is population. For each one Lakh population in rural areas one CHC is set up. Each CHC is set up with the objective of providing standard health services to the public in the rural areas. Accordingly CHC also acts as referral unit in rural areas. Each CHC has 30 beds. Operationalisation of CHC requires expenditure of Rs 20 lakh approximately towards the cost of equipment / infrastructure and salary etc. At present in the state there are 308 CHCs operational. As per July 1987 to March 1997 standards six Specialities were required at CHC level viz. Physician, Surgery,

Gynecologist, Pediatrics, Radiologist and Dental Doctor. The standard was revised and as per March, 1997 to May 1999, seven Specialties were required at CHC levels which were Physician, Surgery, Gynecologist, Dental Doctor, and Pathologist. At present as per standard laid from May, 1999 following five specialties are required at CHC – Physician, Surgery, Gynecologist, Nishchetak, Radiologist.

Level 3

At the third level Health Services are provided in Remote Rural areas through the Primary Health Centres, Additional Primary Health Centres and Sub Centre. PHCs/ Additional PHCs are established level at the village level, having four beds each.

There are presently 1,85,65 sub-centres, 810 Block level PHCs and 2830 additional PHCs operational. Basically mainly Mother and Child care programme is implemented using Sub Centre. Apart from these there are few rural women hospitals where safe delivery facility is provided. Around 20,000/- subcentres on 5000 village population are functioning manned by ANMs

The department is coordinating the implementation of National Health Programme in each district. Important programmes like Family Planning, Immunisation, Malaria eradication, Prevention from AIDS, Filaria eradication, Blindness control, and Iodine Deficiency Disorders being run and monitored by the department officials. The department also provides medical facilities in hospitals created in Police Jails, Central Prisons and PAC. In all, there are 4304 medical units in the state providing the above services with a total bed strength of 53,247.

USAID assisted SIFPSA and World Bank funded AIDS Control society are also functioning to augment Family Welfare and Reproductive Child Health CFW and RCH and AIDS programme.

Uttar Pradesh Health Systems Development Project (UPHSDP) is also working in the state with commitment to improve the delivery system through institutional and human resource development initiatives and to build partnerships in order to provide high quality, affordable, accountable, responsive and integrated healthcare in the state of Uttar Pradesh.

X (a) Organisational Structure of Public Health Sector in Uttar Pradesh

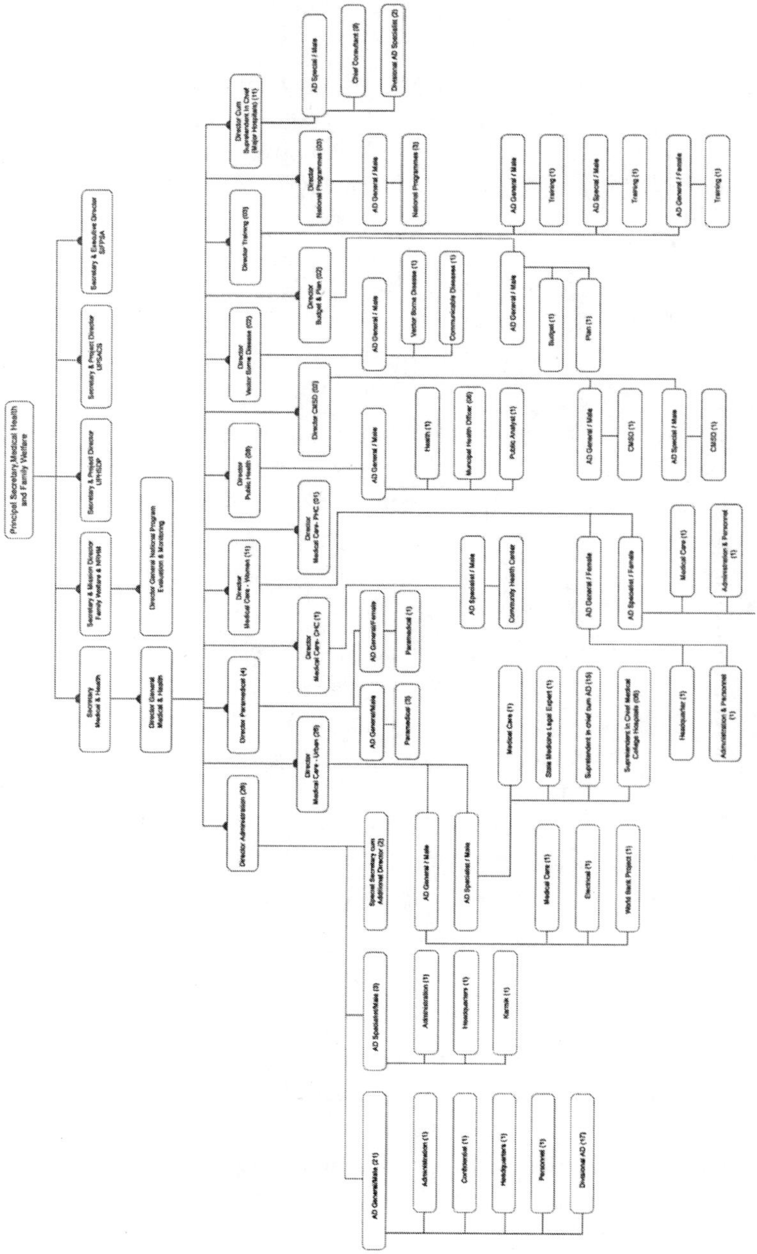

Regional Organisational Structure

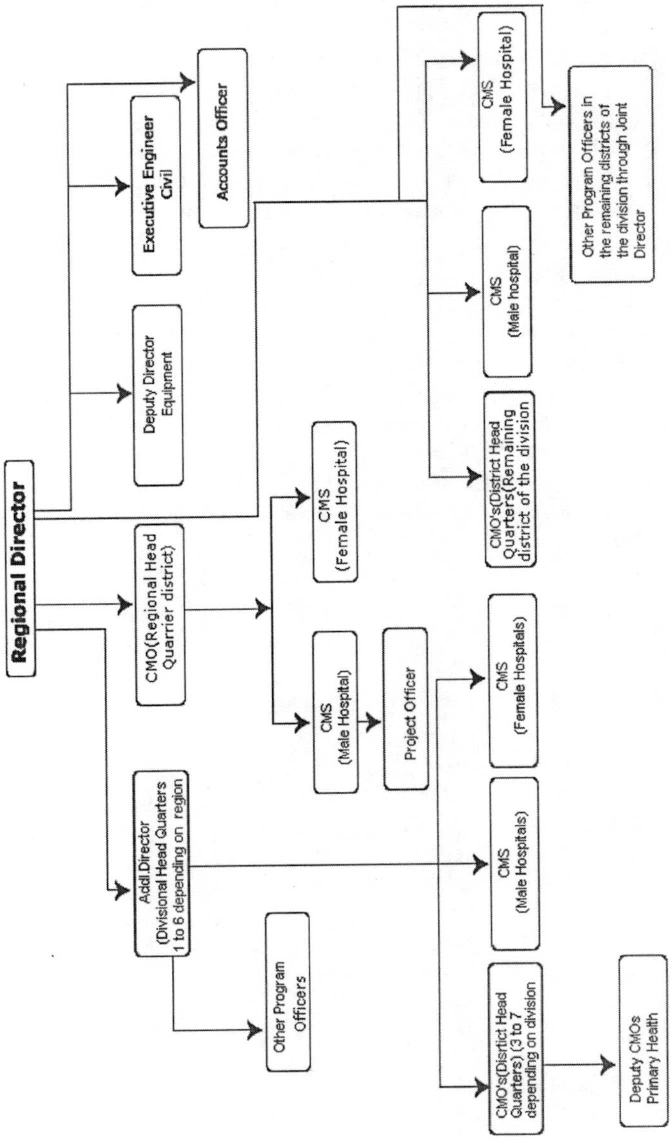

Work Cited

Department of Medicine (2010): "Introduction and Basic Information", Medicine and Health Care, *Government of Uttar Pradesh, website- govup.ac.in*

Dilip T.R. (2002): "Understanding Levels of Morbidity and Hospitalisation in Kerala, India". *Bulletin of the World Health Organisation 2002, 80 (9).*

Division of Economics and Statistics (2008): *Statistical Diary of Uttar Pradesh,* State Planning Institute, Department of Planning, Lucknow.

Division of Economics and Statistics (2009-10): *Arthik Sameeksha,* State Planning Institute, Department of Planning, Lucknow.

Government of Uttar Pradesh (2010): *Profile of Uttar Pradesh,* Government of Uttar Pradesh, website- govup.ac.in

Gupta I (2009): "Potential Impact on Health and Economic Inequality from Cardiovascular Diseases and Diabetes in India: Evidence From the National Sample Survey". *Discussion Paper Series No. 136/2009.*

International Institute for Population Sciences (IIPS) and Macro International (2008): "National Family Health Survey (NFHS-3), India, 2005- 06: Uttar Pradesh" IIPS, Mumbai.

International Institute for Population Sciences (IIPS) and Macro International (2008): "National Family Health Survey (NFHS-3), India, 2005- 06." IIPS, Mumbai.

National Sample Survey Organisation Reports on Various Rounds.

Planning Commission (2008): "Report of the Study Group for Preparation of a Roadmap for Rapid Economic Development of Uttar Pradesh" *Government of India,* New Delhi.

Singh K Ajit (2000): *Uttar Pradesh Development Report 2000,* New Royal Book Company, Lucknow.

State Planning Department (2007): *Human Development Report 2007,* Government of Uttar Pradesh, Lucknow.

Wagstaff A, Paci P, Joshi H (2001): "Causes of Inequality in Health: Who You Are? Where You Live? Or Who Your Parents Were". *Policy Research Working Paper, 2713, World Bank, Washington, DC*

Chapter 4

Inequality in Access to Public Health Care Services in UP

In the health literature three major forms of inequalities have been largely recognised for the persistent and ever widening differential in access and health outcomes. These are historical inequalities, socio-economic inequalities and inequalities in provision and access to health services. Besides other forms of inequality one which is most important and prerequisite for good health is access to healthcare (Baru *et al.* 2010, Krishanan, 1999). In the health literature access has been widely defined as timely utilisation of healthcare services. But to have a complete depiction of public healthcare delivery one needs to deduce utilisation patterns in relation to locational or geographical access, economic or financial access and social access of services (Baru *et al* 2010; Peter *et al* 2008; Krishnan, 1999). Present study documents this broader perspective of provision and access to public health services where in locational or geographical access has been taken as physical availability of public health centres and doctors, economic or financial accessibility as the affordability of healthcare services and social accessibility as the acceptability and utilisation of healthcare services. Uttar Pradesh reflects all kinds of inequalities in its most glaring form as a large number of people share a small chunk of resources. Therefore regional as well as socio-economic inequality is persistent in all the sector of UP in general. But for the present work we have taken up health sector alone with an assumption that it is the prerequisite for equality and development in all other sectors. Thus, this chapter seeks to examine the status of availability of public health services in four regions of Uttar Pradesh. Consequently, it seeks to examine the inequality in context of affordability of healthcare services in terms of cost and burden of healthcare in four economic region of the state and the relative inequality within these regions on the basis of background characteristics of individuals. In continuation to the above two sections the third section looks at the inequality in terms of acceptability and utilisation of healthcare services. Finally, the fourth section provides the rationale for looking at inequality in terms of availability, affordability and acceptability and utilisation of public healthcare services.

The present work basically juxtaposes the supply and demand side of healthcare services. The supply side is captured by the availability of public healthcare centres and health personnel. The demand for healthcare is of two types – one for in-patient treatment and the other is out-patient treatment i.e. mainly clinic and dispensary treatment. Therefore, for demand side analysis we have taken affordability for the out-patient treatment expenditure and for acceptability and utilisation of health services we have taken outpatient and inpatient admission, ANC and vaccination coverage.

I. Availability of Public Health Services and Health Infrastructure

Public healthcare is the provisioning of healthcare facilities by the government. To look at provisioning of public healthcare we are exploring the availability of health centres, availability of human resources at the centres and whether the centre is well equipped with the necessary drugs and other important medical equipments, water and power in particular. In order to evaluate the public health provisioning in the state it is first important to look at the public provisioning of healthcare services i.e. supply side of healthcare services as it extensively affect the pattern and magnitude of demand for healthcare services of individual owing to their background characteristics. We are interested in looking at the impact of supply side of healthcare services on its utilisation and outcomes on the basis of socio-economic group and their relative conditions among four regions. In other words we are inquisitive to look at the status of same marginalised group in one setting and in different setting. Here difference in setting means the variation in availability of public healthcare services. Information on public health infrastructure and personnel is based on unit data provided by the Facility Survey, 2007-08.

"It is a matter of contemporary fact that health facility in India have collapsed. Public health facilities are close to non-existent and private health services far too few, far too exploitative and focused mainly on the urban areas" (Meeta and Rajivlochan, 2010, p. 41) so as in UP rather in more glaring form. Variations in the availability of public health providers are pronounced in requisites of infrastructure, human resources, bed population ratio, appropriate medical equipments and health institutions among the various regions of the Uttar Pradesh (Figure 1). Uttar Pradesh is one such states already going through severe shortage of health personel and health infrastructure (*cf* Chapter 2). Baru *et.al* (2010) illustrate that Kerala has the best and UP has the worst indicators of health service development and health outcomes. Thus UP bears shortage in public health sector along with unequal distribution of public health institution and infrastructure in its various regions. In terms of availability of public health institutions (any government health facility) Bundelkhand region is having highest percentages of villages (47.97 per cent) where any government health facility is available followed by central, eastern and then western region. Indeed it shows a very alarming condition in terms of average population coverage (Table 1). In all the regions there is huge population pressure on the sub-centres, CHC and PHC and one can imagine the population pressure on tertiary healthcare facility given the fact that there is only one public hospital in a district to provide the referral care to rural as well as urban population. However, recent healthcare policy has focused on the infrastructural development in the state as UP is also one among the high focused states in NRHM and it has enormously increased the number of sub-centres, CHCs and PHCs, especially in the regions which are showing poor health outcomes, like, Eastern UP and Bundelkhand.

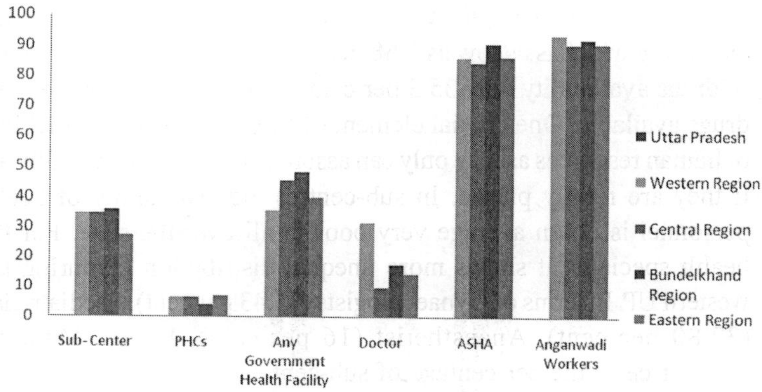

Figure 1: Availabilities of facilities and health personnel in villages by district, Uttar Pradesh, 2007-08.

Table- 1: Average Population Covered by Health Facility by Region UTTAR PRADESH 2007-08

Region	*Sub-centre*	*PHC*	*CHC*
Uttar Pradesh	**8,032**	**69,037**	**176720**
Western Region	7943.65	163133.5	197821.88
Central Region	7634.6	55733.1	165360
Bundelkhand Region	6408.86	30946.86	121043.14
Eastern Region	8447.44	38695.85	187578.56

PHC= Primary Health Centre; CHC= Community Health Centre.

Computed by the author from Unit Data Set of Facility Survey 2007-08.

However, what is particularly important is to have the health personnel in these centres to provide any treatment or medicine. Further analysis shows that most of them are not well equipped. Doctors are not there to treat patients. In this respect it is western UP which is doing better even than the state average. In terms of the availability of doctors 31.37 per cent villages are having doctors in Western UP as opposed to mere 9.64 per cent in Central and 14.27 in Eastern regions. Similarly for Aganwadi workers 93.3 per cent are available in Western UP which is well above the percentage availability in other regions of UP and even to the states average of 91.5 per cent.

In UP on an average only 6.7 per cent sub-centres have regular electricity which is as low as 2.68 per cent in central region. In terms of drugs availability only 35.3 per cent sub-centres have 60 per cent drugs available. One crucial element of healthcare is the availability of human resources as they only can assure consultancy and healthcare if they are rightly placed. In sub-centres the availability of health personnel is on an average very poor in all over the state. For the health specialist it shows more unequal distribution favouring the western UP. In terms of Gynaecologists (35.43 per cent), Paediatrician (37.80 per cent), Anaesthetist (16 per cent), Health Manager (4.2 per cent) the per centage of sub-centres in western UP. is well above the state average and very high in comparison to other regions.

Table 2: Available Infrastructures/Human Resources and Services at Primary Health Centres by Region- UP- 2007-08

	Number of PHC having				
Region	*Uttar Pradesh (per cent)*	*Western Region*	*Central Region*	*Bundel-khand Region*	*Eastern Region*
Medical officer	**652(79.6)**	92.39	82.64	71.84	73.87
Pharmacist	**647(79.0)**	84.77	81.94	63.11	79.20
Functional OT	**365 (44.6)**	79.19	33.33	35.92	33.07
Functioning PHC 24 hours	**373(45.5)**	74.11	44.44	47.57	30.4
At least 4 Beds	**464(56.7)**	85.28	54.17	59.22	41.87
Regular Power Supply	**95(11.6)**	6.60	9.72	22.33	12
Having Functional Vehicle	**148(18.1)**	34.01	22.22	7.77	10.93
Essential drugs (at least 60%)	**447 (54.6)**	77.16	55.56	58.25	41.33
Total Number of PHCs	**819(100.0)**	**197**	**144**	**103**	**375**

Computed by the author from Unit Data Set of Facility Survey 2007- 08.

In UP only 45.5 per cent PHCs are 24 hour functioning, 56.7 per cent have at least 4 beds, only 11.6 per cent have regular power supply and only 18.1 per cent are having functional vehicle. However, western regions of UP is in better position with 74.11 per cent having 24 hour functioning PHCs as against only 30.4 per cent in Eastern region. Similar is the situation with beds availability in these institutions, 85.28 per cent PHCs in western regions are having at least four beds as against just half in eastern region. In terms of functional vehicle the situation is all the more worse in Bundelkhand and eastern region with only 7.77 and 10.93 per cent PHCs having functional vehicle respectively. Still relatively in western UP 34 per cent are having functional vehicle (Table 2).

Further coming to the specific health facility available at PHCs, only 15 per cent PHCs having new born care, even less than 50 per cent having functional OT, only 21.4 per cent having cold chain equipment and approximately half of the PHCs having essential drugs and of all these the higher concentration is in western UP itself and a very small percentage available in central, Bundelkhand and eastern UP. 79.19 per cent functional OT are in western UP as opposed to nearly 34 per cent in central, Bundelkhand and eastern UP. Moreover in some cases the gap is so wide as 73.60 per cent are cold chain equipped in western UP and only 1.6 and 1.94 per cent in eastern and Bundelkhand regions respectively. Further in terms of essential drugs 77.16 per cent PHCs in western region are keeping it as opposed to 41.33 per cent in eastern region and nearly half of the PHCs of Bundelkhand and central regions having essential drugs available at their centre. Same is the case with facility available at sub-centres (Table 3).

Table 3: Human Resources/Services Available at Community Health Centres by Regions

UTTAR PRADESH, 2007-08

Region	*Number of CHC having*				
	Uttar Pradesh (per cent)	*Western Region*	*Central Region*	*Bundel-khand Region*	*Eastern Region*
Obstetric Gynaecologist	**135 (19.5)**	35.43	24.11	13.21	13.17
Paediatrician	**144 (20.8)**	37.80	21.99	13.21	15.59
Anaesthetist	**111 (16)**	25.98	17.02	11.32	12.90
Health Manager	**19 (2.7)**	4.72	2.84	1.89	2.15
Functional OT	**613 (88.5)**	78.74	85.11	84.91	93.55
Total number of CHCs	**693 (100)**	**127**	**141**	**53**	**372**

Computed by the author from Unit Data Set of Facility Survey 2007-08.

Therefore in Bundelkhand and Eastern region what is particularly crucial for the poor health outcomes and access to health services is that in spite of larger number of SCs, PHCs, and CHCs, they are running short of human resources and appropriate medicines (Tables 2 and 3). The building only can't provide health services. Rather, the foremost requisite is medical health personel, appropriate equipment and medicines at affordable prices.

II. Affordability of Public Health Services in UP and regions

Affordability of healthcare services incorporates the direct and indirect cost of treatment and household capacity to meet those costs (Gilison, 2007; Baru *et al* 2010). Affordability is something which is directly linked with the public health provisioning and combined together both may cause equal/ unequal access to healthcare services and health outcome. The public healthcare provisioning certainly reduces the cost of healthcare as government doesn't play with profit motive. Therefore, the group which is economically poor can also have access to care. In fact affordability is linked to many factors of which economic status and active role of the government are crucial elements.

To obtain information for the affordability of healthcare services we have used data from NSS 60th round survey during January-June 2004 of morbidity and utilisation of health services. Here we have taken cost incurred for out-patient[1] treatment in all the four regions and for socio-economic groups within these regions. The total cost of treatment includes not only the direct payments made to the health centres but also the cost of medicines, investigations and tests. It does not presumably include the cost of transportation and boarding and lodging. The ranking are somewhat also altered on the basis of total cost per day of treatment due to the variation in the number of days of treatment in different regions and different socio-economic group.

We have first calculated the average total cost of treatment and its source of financing as the health expenditure cause a huge financial distress for the household. Around 63.22 million individuals or 11.88 million households were pushed to BPL due to healthcare expenditure in 2004 (Berman *et al* 2010). We have tried to look at the relative expenditure on health among the region for different socio-economic group. First we analyses the variation there in and then we move on to the source of financing of this expenditure as it is very crucial to know the impact of health expenditure upon household. We have further made an attempt to estimate the burden of treatment[2] for each region and different socio-economic group based on the information provided by NSS. However, such exercises of estimating burden of treatment is difficult and has its limitations owing to the fact that we do not have data on the income of these different groups. NSS 60th round has also collected information on consumer expenditure. Information on the cost of treatment incurred by people is also given. We have thus estimated total per capita consumer expenditure corresponding to these socio-economic groups from the data on consumer expenditure collected for the same year. The relative burden of treatment is then defined as the ratio of treatment cost to the annual per capita expenditure of the corresponding population of different socio-economic groups.

II a. Health Expenditure and Source of Financing

In UP out of pocket expenditure (OOP) forms a disproportionately large component of total health expenditure. Besides OOP expenditure there are indirect costs involved to this which is loss of income due to the illness. Average total expenditure on consumption of healthcare is higher in western UP (637), followed by eastern (597), central (594) and Bundelkhand region (564). But what is particularly important is the source of financing. The analysis of the data from the NSS 60th round shows that the high burden of expenditure on healthcare, is largely financed through two major sources: 1. household's own resources and 2. borrowings. In Bundelkhand region close to nine per cent of the health expenses for outpatient care is financed through borrowings, which is the highest in comparison to the other regions of UP. Further in central and Bundelkhand region approximately four per cent expenses are financed through contributions (Table 4). However, the corresponding expenditure

Table 4: Distribution of Expenditure by Source of Finance

	Average Total Expenditure	*Household Income/ Saving*	*Expenses Borrowings*	*Percentage Borrowed*	*Average Total Expenditure*	*Household Income/ Saving*	*Expenses Borrowings*	*Percentage Borrowed*
		Western				**Central**		
	637.79	**596.66**	**1112.85**	**8.09**	**594.05**	**589.14**	**2081.01**	**4.66**
Religion								
Hindu	671.849	633.88	1086.65	8.89	584.07	587.25	2276.77	4.48
Muslim	508.52	475.13	1251.81	5.47	641.69	596.45	1453.68	5.39
Differential	163.329	158.75	-165.16	3.42	-57.62	-9.2	823.09	-0.91
Social Group								
Scheduled caste	590.14	614.97	744.72	11.21	466.83	456.51	608.01	7.46
Others	748.6	674.51	1385.57	5.66	786.45	827.76	4683.36	3.13
Differential	-158.46	-59.54	-640.85	5.55	-319.62	-371.25	-4075.35	4.32
Sector								
Rural	616.69	607.71	1050.67	9.44	598.99	598.99	1554.03	8.39
Urban	676.24	574.62	1329.53	5.40	583.43	583.43	854.72	3.48
Differential	-59.55	33.09	-278.86	4.04	15.56	15.56	699.31	4.91
MPCE-Class								
300- 600	509.83	516.24	940.15	9.28	554.86	554.86	1828	8.03
900 & above	1149.45	1019.2	2959.85	5.16	786	786	7750	0.67
Differential	-639.62	-502.96	-2019.7	4.12	-231.14	-231.14	-5922	7.37

(Cond...)

	Eastern				Southern			
	597.15	652.46	1555.58	5.72	564.66	557.85	856.47	8.73
Religion								
Hindu	614.8	688.77	1678.89	6.24	573.51	573.08	886.56	8.47
Muslim	532.2	505.01	692.39	3.62	444.1	403.67	630.75	11.43
Differential	82.6	183.76	986.5	2.62	129.41	169.41	255.81	-2.96
Social Group								
Scheduled caste	589.48	595.64	1099.35	8.97	606.4	503.98	471.94	17.34
Others	622.32	616.23	644.81	4.55	731.26	824.46	1412.83	9.58
Differential	-32.84	-20.59	454.54	4.43	-124.86	-320.48	-940.89	7.75
Sector								
Rural	610.39	610.39	994.4	7.11	626.68	626.68	652.52	10.98
Urban	544.63	544.63	1304	4.03	488.56	488.56	748.71	4.96
Differential	65.76	65.76	-309.6	3.08	138.12	138.12	-96.19	6.02
MPCE-Class								
300- 600	538.85	538.85	1080.53	6.00	508.45	508.45	692.45	11.76
900 & above	916.61	916.61	2139.5	8.77	692.73	692.73	2000	2.94
Differential	-377.76	-377.76	-1058.97	-2.77	-184.28	-184.28	-1307.55	8.82

Computed by the author from NSS 60th round- 2004.

in terms of hospitalisation has not been incorporated in present analysis which is much higher in the state as such (Baru *et al* 2010).

Adverse socio-economic differential in average total expenditure is a situation wide spread in all regions of UP, but the situation is the worst in Bundelkhand region in particular. The regional variation in socio- economic differential in health expenditure is exhibited from the fact that the average expenditure on health is very low among the Muslims than their Hindu counterparts, especially the gap is higher in eastern UP (183.76) followed by Bundelkhand UP (169.41). Similar is the case among various caste groups. Here the gap in average expenditure is higher in central followed by Bundelkhand regions. Similar is the case with economic group and rural urban sector where inequality is the highest in Bundelkhand region. Here the linkage between public health provisioning and inequality among socio-economic group can be well established. The western region with well-equipped public health system has low socio-economic inequality than the eastern and Bundelkhand regions.

Further, borrowing is one of the important sources of health expenditure financing of the household. However, the gap is not very sharp by the religious background, that means both the major religious group, Hindu and Muslim, fall upon borrowings for financing their health expenditure. For social group the situation is very bad for SCs relative to their general counterpart in all over the state in general but in particular the situation is very worst in Bundelkhand with wide gap of -7.76 between SC and General castes group. However, it is nearly close to five per cent in western UP and a bit lower in central and eastern regions. It is worth mentioning that the low expenditure does not mean higher affordability or lack of diseases. Rather, the group may not be in the ambit of formal healthcare providers or lack of awareness or lack of facility may be responsible for lack of demand and low expenditure. This conclusion may be arrived at after having a close examination of the availability of public health infrastructure and services among the four regions. That an individual with poor background in terms of socio-religious group or income has better access to health facility and consequently good health outcome in western region than in any other region of the state. Thus, looking at the source of funding, the borrowings are systematically high among the Muslims in all regions and the SCs sub-groups. The socio-economic inequality in terms of affordability of public healthcare services is particularly highest in Bundelkhand region, followed by western and eastern region.

Here we have taken household health expenditure as proxy of their demand and access to healthcare services and assumed that the group with less average expenditure has low demand for healthcare services. It can be clearer by the individual reporting about why they did not seek healthcare. As this is something more close to acceptability of healthcare services it has been discussed at length in next section, where the major disadvantaged group reported financial reason as a main cause of not accessing public healthcare.

Table 5: Burden of Treatment

Region/Background Characteristics	*Western*	*Central*	*Eastern*	*Bundelkhand*
Sector				
Rural	17.84	22.64	20.72	21.79
Urban	14.03	13.55	12.30	14.85
Religion				
Hindu	17.11	18.63	19.69	19.16
Muslim	13.00	20.16	14.75	13.53
Social Group				
SC	19.35	20.50	24.54	23.99
OBC	15.94	16.28	18.69	14.83
General	15.03	19.50	15.60	18.39
MPCE Class				
0-300	19.50	25.01	19.84	23.55
300-600	16.54	21.27	18.70	18.97
600-900	14.30	19.12	21.25	18.75
900 & Above	17.46	12.17	13.38	15.06
Total	**16.15**	**18.81**	**18.67**	**18.57**

Computed by the Author from Unit Data Set of 'NSS 60th round – 2004.

II (b) Burden of Treatment

The burden of treatment is not the same as the cost of treatment. The burden of treatment will depend on the nature and duration of illness, individual or family income, external sources of financing like health insurance or employer support and the loss of income of the patient and others during the period of illness (Krishnan, 1999). We define the burden of treatment for an individual or family as the ratio of the total cost of illness to the income of the individual or family.

Explicitly the relative burden of treatment is the lowest in western region, even well below the other region of the state i.e. Central, Eastern and Bundelkhand bearing almost equal burden of treatment. This measure, however, varies widely across socio-economic group among the four regions. These measure are given in Figs. 2, 3, 4 and 5 for socio-economic group among the four region –

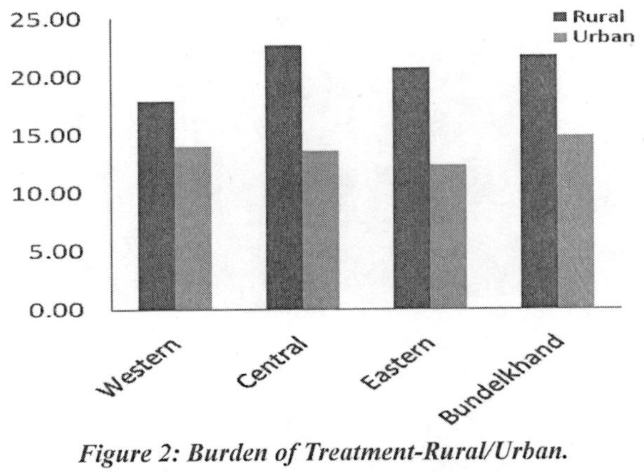

Figure 2: Burden of Treatment-Rural/Urban.

It is interesting to note that it is rural, poor and marginalised section of society who is the worst sufferer in terms of burden of treatment, regardless of the region he/she may belong to. One exception to this is that in central and Bundelkhand region households from general caste are bearing higher burden of treatment than OBC households, yet it is well below the burden of treatment born by the SC sub-group. Indeed one can see a massive variation in inequality

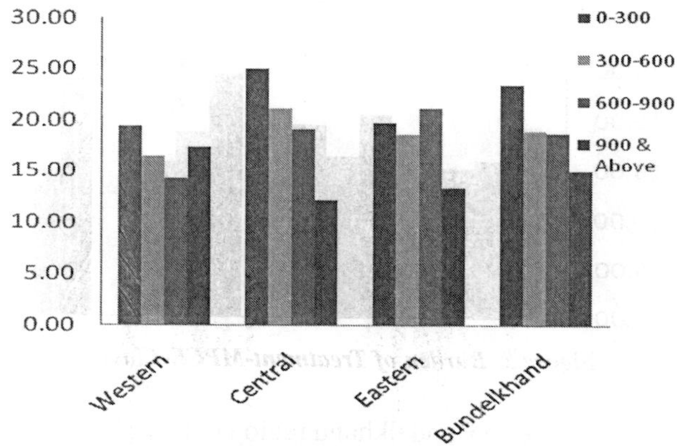

Figure 3: Burden of Treatment-MPCE-Class.

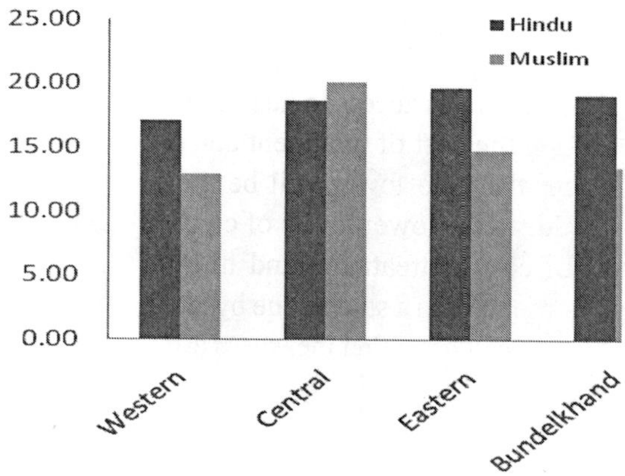

Figure 4: Burden of Treatment-Hindu/Muslim.

on the basis of socio-economic characteristics among these four regions. With respect to socio-economic inequality it is the highest in Bundelkhand region followed by eastern UP and central UP (Figures 2, 3, 4, and 5). Following the above analysis and explanation it can easily be concluded that socio-economic inequality in terms of burden of treatment is always lower in western UP. That means a household belongs to rural area or a poor or SC belonging to western region always have a lower burden of treatment than a comparable

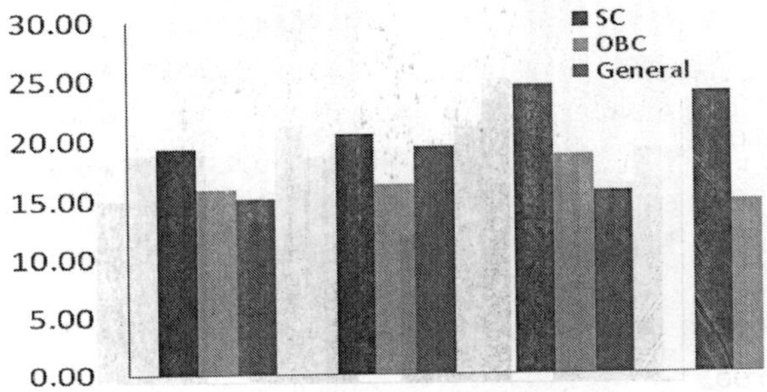

Figure 5: Burden of Treatment-MPCE-Class

household belonging to Bundelkhand region or to certain extent from eastern region too. From here it can also be inferred that these group have much more equal opportunity of access to healthcare services and better chances of survival in western UP than their counterparts from Bundelkhand and eastern region. The burden of treatment can be a major determinant of access to health services as it is something directly reflecting the cost of treatment and household's capacity to afford it. Higher the ratio lower will be the household capacity to bear it. Either due to the lower levels of consumption expenditure or higher levels of cost of treatment and in both the situation it is a setback for a household. In a study done by Krishnan (1999) he argues that "if we were to calculate Sen measures of index of poverty before and after treatment, then the degree of poverty would have gone up in the case of these groups of the population (p. 224)" and obviously poverty would have specifically shoot up in Bundelkhand and eastern region as well the magnitude of inequality. He also argues that in case of households below the poverty line, treatment costs would have almost definitely led to a reduction in calorie intake, not only for the person treated but also for other members of the household. Such a reduction in food intake could increase the risk to infection and the level of morbidity in society.

Moreover on the basis of above analysis it can be undoubtedly demonstrated that the burden of treatment are closely linked to provisioning of public healthcare services. The burden of treatment is high in those regions where public health infrastructure is least developed, for example, in Bundelkhand region where public provisioning of healthcare services is not in good shape the infrastructural development in terms of increased number of PHCs, CHCs and Sub-centres could not make any dent to the cost of care as they are lacking in health personnel, required equipment and necessary medicine and therefore burden of treatment is high in Bundelkhand.

III. Acceptability and Utilisation of Public Health Services in UP and regions

Besides availability and affordability of health services the third element in access to health is the acceptability of the public healthcare services. It is the social and cultural distance between healthcare systems and their uses. It incorporates quality care along with faith in public health system. Since acceptability of healthcare services is not directly measurable it can only be identified through the utilisation pattern of healthcare services and the willingness to buy healthcare services.

To obtain information on utilisation of healthcare services we utilised data from NSS 60th round. The information used for the analysis is whether the treatment taken on medical advice or not and then whether the medical advice taken are from government sources or otherwise. To have deeper analysis we have taken few more indicators like OPD- patient (male and female), inpatient admitted (male and female) and utilisation of public services for the morbidity (fever and diarrhoea) treatment of children. The data source for these are unit data of facility survey and RCH unit data of married women conducted in 2007- 08. However, the socio-economic variation cannot be brought into analysis due to the unavailability of background characteristics of these individuals.

The analysis brings into light the fairly low utilisation of government health services across the four regions of Uttar Pradesh, both in rural and urban areas and among the various socio-economic groups. This is broadly supported by other studies too. However, most of these studies are at aggregate level i.e. on state or country level (Prabhu, 1999; Baru *et al* 2010).

In UP nearly 20 per cent of the population does not seek formal care. They don't consider their diseases to be serious or took some tablets on casual suggestions or from medical shops due to lack of awareness or willingness. A large proportion doesn't go to the government health providers to seek care, only close to sixteen per cent availed the health facility from any public health institution. In western UP, nearly 87.6 per cent are seeking care on medical advice; well above the state average and relatively very high from other regions. However, their proportion in seeking care from government health facility is the lowest among the four regions of the state. As opposed to this in Bundelkhand and eastern region, where a very small percentage of people are seeking care on medical advice, a larger number are going to do so from public health facility. Now this can be well connected to the higher average health expenditure in western region as they seek care from high cost health providers combined with higher degree of urbanisation, economic development and educational achievement of this region. As opposed to this in eastern and Bundelkhand regions, relatively backward regions of the state with higher incidence of poverty, a larger percentage does not go to seek care at all and those who do so are mostly going to public health providers (Table 6). Therefore, it is all the more important, especially for the poor and marginalised, that public healthcare system be strong enough to provide universal healthcare to all. Indeed the low quality care is indicative from the fact that eastern and Bundelkhand are the two regions with relatively poor health outcomes than other regions of the state. Thus, mere existence of public health facility doesn't guarantee good health outcomes.

In terms of socio-economic differential Muslims are worse off relative to Hindus in seeking formal healthcare. A higher percentage of Muslims seek informal treatment either from medical shops, quacks or others suggestions (Table 6). Again in terms of caste category lower caste people are more dependent on public healthcare services or they go without care. As against this the people from general caste are more reluctant to seek care from public health providers. Generally they seek care from high cost private health providers, as nearly

Table 6

	Treatment Taken on Medical Advice				**Utilisation of Government Hospitals**			
Region	**Western**	**Central**	**Eastern**	**Southern**	**Western**	**Central**	**Eastern**	**Southern**
	87.6	77.18	76.82	76.19	11.86	21.56	16.01	26.34
Religion								
Hindu	97.22	93.81	95.46	92.29	11.13	23.63	17.62	25.89
Muslim	93.58	93.64	88.98	100	12	7.89	10.23	30.48
Differential	**3.64**	**0.17**	**6.48**	**-7.71**	**-0.87**	**15.74**	**7.39**	**-4.59**
Caste								
Scheduled caste	98.06	93.37	98.27	90.09	12.18	29.93	20.11	30.77
Others	95.65	93.74	89.3	97.44	10.71	22.74	19.37	30.49
Differential	**2.41**	**-0.37**	**8.97**	**-7.35**	**1.47**	**7.19**	**0.74**	**0.28**
Sector								
Rural	87.42	70.36	75.39	60.73	10.14	20.42	15	31.51
Urban	88.02	90.4	83.09	77.3	15.58	24.27	13.36	22.31
Differential	**-0.6**	**-20.04**	**-7.7**	**-16.57**	**-5.44**	**-3.85**	**1.64**	**9.2**
MPCE-Class								
300- 600	88.24	72.84	75.84	60.25	9.42	20.09	14.18	30.94
900 & above	90.04	91.62	82.73	86.84	14.89	24.48	16.36	21.21
Differential	**-1.8**	**-18.78**	**-6.89**	**-26.59**	**-5.47**	**-4.39**	**-2.18**	**9.73**

Computed by the author from NSS 60th round- 2004.

95 per cent of people from the better of group reported taking healthcare on medical advice.

Further analysis of the data shows that inequalities in terms of seeking care on medical advice is present in most glaring form in Bundelkhand and eastern region with wide gap of 7.71 and 6.48, respectively. The similar kind of pattern can be seen with caste category. In general and SC the gap in seeking formal care is very high in Bundelkhand with the difference of 7.35 per cent. However, in other regions too such kind of inequality is present but not as wide as in Bundelkhand and eastern regions. Further, in the utilisation of healthcare services on the basis of religion and social group a major variation can be seen among the four regions of the state. Here again the inequality is high in Bundelkhand and eastern regions. However, in terms of utilisation of government health services the inequality is the highest in central region in all socio-economic groups.

It is persistently brought out in the analysis that the inequality is very low in western region. This is partly because of it being a richer region. Rather, what we notice is that absolute number of public health institutions is low in western UP as compared to other regions, but most of them are well equipped and better performing in terms of meeting healthcare needs of the relatively worse off group of the society.

Of course, it also emerges from analysis that a large percentage of people seek care from private providers in western UP, as very large percentage of individuals are seeking care on medical advice but a very low proportion goes to avail facility from public health institutions. Therefore, it is not only the physical existence of public health institution, but the well functioning institutions are, to larger extent, responsible for low level of inequality in western UP. As opposed to this Bundelkhand and eastern regions are already backward regions with less functional and adverse infrastructure in the public health institution, which on the one hand increases the burden given the small resources available and on the other hand provides a very small cake to share in larger number. As a result inequality increases with better off taking away the benefits.

The malfunctioning of public health provisioning in backward region of the state is clear from the fact that the number of OPD patient male as well as female in CHC is the highest in western region denoting greater utilisation and acceptance of health services. As against this it is the lowest in eastern region (898.24), followed by Bundelkhand region (981.90) even below the state average. In western UP the inpatient admissions of male are just double the eastern region. The same story is repeated in a more glaring form in case of PHCs also. The persistent regional inequality exhibits from the fact that only one-fourth of OPD patient male and female are there in eastern and Bundelkhand region. However, central UP is in better position near to the states average in comparison to these two regions. In terms of inpatient admission the differential is as wide as 19.04 per cent male and 32.11 per cent female are admitted in western region as oppose to 1.72 per cent male and 2.30 per cent female in eastern region have utilised public health institutions for hospitalisation. Similar is the situation of Bundelkhand region. Here also the central UP is doing better than the two regions of Bundelkhand and eastern

Table 7: Utilisation of Public Health Institution

CHC	*Western*	*Central*	*Bundel-khand*	*Eastern*	*Total*
OPD patient - male	1498.29	1330	981.9	898.24	1055.49
OPD patient - female	1495.35	1187.32	1022.45	808.76	989.1
Inpatient admissions - Male	44.67	33.15	54.59	20.86	26.57
Inpatient admissions - Female	66.05	60.23	96.93	58.66	61.7
PHC					
OPD patient - male	778.01	430.6	237	264.56	400.77
OPD patient - female	861.49	349.99	189.5	260.62	392.83
Inpatient admissions - Male	19.04	17.24	2.98	1.72	8.63
Inpatient admissions - Female	32.11	19.08	3.4	2.3	12.35

Computed by the author from Unit Data Set of Facility Survey 2007-08.

UP. In general the utilisation of public health facility is poor all over the state but situation gets more alarming when we look at it through regional variation and locate socio-economic groups in these regions (Table 7). However inequality in reference to background characteristics can't be measured for inpatient and OPD patient due to the lack of information about the socio-economic status of these people. But such a low level of utilisation of public health facility in Bundelkhand and eastern region is indicative of worse off going without the healthcare. The people who are not under the ambit of relatively cheaper public health services can't go to avail facility through private health providers who are there for making profit.

The utilisation of service for treatment of children for acute respiratory tract infection is generally very low in UP with only 6.28 per cent children treated for diarrhoea and only 7.99 per cent got treatment for acute respiratory tract infection. However, it is quite better in western UP (10.99) as opposed to a worse situation in Bundelkhand region (2.92). In such a situation it can be easily guessed that those small percentages must be a section of population who are on higher or middle hierarchy of societal system. It is just because the fact that whenever there is a small piece to be shared it is better off who corner out most of the gains. Similarly, in immunisation of infant and children the percentage in western region is just double the central region, triple the eastern region and four times higher than the Bundelkhand region (Table 8).

Table 8

Region	*Summary of number of children treated for diarrhea*	*Summary of number of children treated for acute respiratory tract infection*	*Summary of number of infants and children immunized*
Western Region	5.69	10.99	148.51
Central Region	8.96	6.91	78.11
Bundelkhand Region	4.12	2.92	33.65
Eastern Region	5.47	7.61	58.13
Total	**6.28**	**7.99**	**83.55**

Computed by the Author from Unit Data Set of Facility Survey – 2007- 08.

IV. Access to Healthcare Services and its Consequences upon Health Outcomes

In order to have more explicit picture of public healthcare delivery it is important to look at availability, affordability and acceptability and utilisation of healthcare services in relation to health outcomes. Since measuring health outcomes has various limitations of subjectivity where in marginalised and poor seem to enjoying good health outcomes and therefore it can be wrongly inferred that they are enjoying better access to healthcare services too. A detailed analysis of this phenomenon is required in order to arrive at any conclusion. Therefore, before establishing the link between accesses to healthcare services and health outcomes, we need to have a tribulations in measuring health outcomes. For the analysis of this section we have been relied on data from two sources, namely NSS and NFHS. For acute, chronic and undiagnosed diseases we have taken data from NSS 60th round. It provides data for number of disease for the 15 days of recall period. The details are given for all members of household who fell ill during the last 15 days. Then for Asthma and Diabetes we have taken data from NFHS-3.

V. Tribulations in Measuring Health Outcomes

For the analysis of this section we have been relied on data from various sources like for acute, chronic and undiagnosed diseases we have taken data from NSS 60th round. It provides data for number of disease for the 15 days of recall period the details are given for all the members of household who fell ill during the last 15 days. Then for Asthma and Diabetes we have taken data from NFHS-3.

Inequality in health manifests itself into subjective and objective indicators. Inequalities based on subjective indicators are never captured fully, especially from indicators like morbidity (incidence of sickness). It tends to be very higher for objective indicators of ill health like malnutrition and mortality. It is often noted that measures for the incidence of sickness sometimes produce wicked gradients with the better off reporting worse health than the poor (Table 9).

Table 9: Inequality in Actual and Self Assessed Health

Background Characteristics	*Acute Disease*	*Chronic Disease*	*Un Diag-nosed*	*Asthma Men*	*Asthma Women*	*Diabetes Men*	*Diabetes Women*	*Under-Five Mortality*
Religion								
Hindu	4.86	4.36	0.22					115.8
Muslim	4.5	3.64	0.13					101.1
Location								
Rural	4.4	3.89	0.21	1376	1153	383	270	116.9
Urban	6.2	5.59	0.17	882	904	623	709	94.8
Castes								
SC	3.44	3.09	0.3					135.1
OBC	4.46	4.31	0.2					111
General	6.84	5.25	0.12					87.7
Level of Education								
Illiterate	4.08	3.41	0.19	1919	1414	453	276	124.3
Some education	5.1	4.61	0.23	2014	1727	375	290	
Higher Education	7.03	7.18	0.1	900	606	689	816	58.5
Gender								
Male	12.4	14.23	2.34					100.9
Female	9.37	11.08	0.39					124.7
Wealth Index								
Lowest /0-300	2.72	2.48	0.11	58	48	2334	908	135.4
Middle /300-600	4.83	3.99	0.24	314	374	1126	1224	114.9
Fourth/600-900	5.68	5.29	0.2	635	509	827	959	84
Highest /900 & above	7.64	8.23	0.13	1015	889	708	754	61.8

Source: Values for Chronic, Acute and Undiagnosed- computed by the Author, Asthma, Diabetes and Under-5 Mortality, IIPS Macro International-2007.

Morbidity or feeling sick is a subjective phenomenon and its measurement is characterised by conceptual limitations like lack of awareness, adaptive preferences or lack of health facilities for the diagnosis of the diseases. That is why the concrete evidence of a relation between mortality and morbidity is lacking; regions with higher morbidity are reported to have lower mortality and vice versa (Dilip, 2002). Therefore, it is difficult to establish the relationship between public healthcare and health outcomes especially with indicators like morbidity.

While better off groups report higher morbidity, worse of group, not so aware of their sickness even if they are in their worse of health status, report lower morbidity. This is corroborated by the fact that the poor and the lower castes reported higher for the commonly known diseases and diseases with visible symptoms like asthma, whereas there is very less reporting for the diseases which require awareness, knowledge and diagnosis like diabetes (Table 9). For diabetes the reporting by this group is negligible, indicative of lack of awareness, lack of accessibility or affordability of health services.

On an average 105 persons per thousand have reported any kind of ailment in Uttar Pradesh in 60th NSS round, far less than Kerala's reported morbidity of 205. Low life expectancy for men and women both, coupled with high death rate in Uttar Pradesh also reflects underreporting of ailments and ignorance of diseases or perception differences on the part of disadvantaged group resulting into a greater toll of death in silence. As a matter of fact UP has quite higher infant death rate of 70 in comparison to the national average of 55 and ranked 13th among major fifteen states of India. This could be the case in UP as household spends Rs 17158 crore on health which is 92.2 per cent of all health expenditure, whereas government spends only Rs 2650 crore. In Kerala, the household sector spends only Rs 8373 crore, while in Tamil Nadu household sector spends Rs.3624 crore only.

All indicators of early childhood mortality in UP are not only higher than national average but neonatal mortality, postnatal mortality and infant mortality is more than double of national average, child mortality is more than five times of national average and under five mortality is more than three times of national average. In all indicators urban UP is better than rural UP Interestingly, probability of survival of Muslim child is always better than Hindu child. All mortality rates are always higher in rural area and Hindu religious group. A child of a SC mother has lower chance of survival than any other caste groups. Wealth appears to improve child survival chances across all mortality rates. Here the education of women plays a very substantial role as the child survival chances of an educated mother (of ten or more years of schooling) are very high as compared to an uneducated mother (Table 9). Looking at the Table 10 few important facts appear, like there is some kind of underreporting of ailment by the poor which can be a result of either the lack of knowledge and awareness or unavailability of health facilities. To examine this question the indicator of objective health outcome (like CMR, under five mortality, infant mortality, death rate, and life expectancy, or the medically examined morbidity[3]) among various socio-economic groups has also been taken. The justification behind taking objective health indicator is that inequality in health is almost always to the disadvantage of poor, rural class and women. They suffer from multiplicity of deprivations and that translates into bad health and premature deaths (Gupta, 2009; Wagstaff, 2001).

VI. Linking Access to Healthcare Services to Health Outcomes

This section utilises data again from NSS 60th round for individual ailment during the last 15 days of survey. It also uses data for CMR from SRS and data for fever and diarrhoea is taken from DLHS-3 for married women.

The improved healthcare facilities and higher affordability and utilisation of public healthcare services are responsible for better health outcomes in any region. The reporting of ailment, Diarrhoea and ARI among children is persistently high in western UP, while it is consistently very low in eastern and Bundelkhand regions. Here an interesting thing to point out is that the higher morbidity reporting region has the lower CMR (Table 10). Now it can be well inferred that the inadequate and poorly equipped public health infrastructure jeopardises access to health from several sides like reducing the affordability of healthcare services among the poor population, increasing the cost of healthcare service by providing space to private providers and underutilisation of services, which in combination results into bad health outcome along with increased inequality among the region. The very good example of such a case is eastern and Bundelkhand region of UP where the average health expenditure is relatively high along with underutilisation of public health services and these are the region with worse health outcomes.

Table 10: Incidence of Ailment and CMR

State/Region	*Acute Ailment*	*Chronic Ailment*	*Children Suffered from Diarrhea*	*Children Suffered from ARI*	*CMR-2001*
Uttar Pradesh	25.8	20.64	16.2	16.9	95.69
Western	32.67	25.19	19.37	20.99	90.69
Central	28.19	21.08	14.67	16.99	95.9
Eastern	18.27	16.55	11.17	12.11	104.57
Southern	25.53	17.87	12.65	11.71	91.59

Acute Ailment includes-

Chronic Ailment includes-

Note: Table based on women with youngest living children born since 01.01.2004.

Source: Computed by Author from Unit Data Set of NSS 60th Round.

The table below shows that the Bundelkhand and eastern regions holds highest inequality in terms of reporting of acute and chronic ailment between Hindus and Muslims and between SC and general castes (Table 11). The inequality in Bundelkhand is exceptionally very high in religious group, it is 8.29 for acute ailment and 11.02 for chronic ailment. Similar kind of result can be seen for other ailment like diarrhoea and fever among the children (Table 11).

Table 11: Socio-economic Variation in Reporting of Ailment within the Region

	Acute Ailment				*Chronic Ailment*			
Religion	*Western*	*Central*	*Eastern*	*Southern*	*Western*	*Central*	*Eastern*	*Southern*
Hindu	32.97	28.29	17.75	26.19	25.06	21.16	15.68	17
Muslim	31.65	27.8	21.18	17.9	25.64	20.77	21.52	28.02
Differential	**1.32**	**0.49**	**-3.43**	**8.29**	**-0.58**	**0.39**	**-5.84**	**-11.02**
Caste								
Scheduled caste	34.05	26.91	16.7	23.97	22.8	19.6	15.37	23.2
Others	30.5	27.11	19.18	28.55	28.48	24.98	19.52	21.1
Differential	3.55	-0.2	-2.48	-4.58	-5.68	-5.38	-4.15	2.1

(Contd...)

Sector								
Rural	35.52	30.61	18.56	26.49	24.01	20.68	16.22	16.09
Urban	27.31	22.62	16.63	23.97	27.41	21.99	18.38	20.76
Differential	**8.21**	**7.99**	**1.93**	**2.52**	**-3.4**	**-1.31**	**-2.16**	**-4.67**
MPCE Class								
300- 600	39.92	33.19	20.78	29.95	25.31	24.14	18.27	21.43
900 & above	25.64	19.33	19.13	20.69	35.29	32.33	23.83	22.99
Differential	**14.28**	**13.86**	**1.65**	**9.26**	**-9.98**	**-8.19**	**-5.56**	**-1.56**

	Diarrhea				**Fever**			
Religion	Western	Central	Eastern	Southern	Western	Central	Eastern	Southern
Hindu	14.09	11.06	7.15	6.7	19.79	15.55	12.75	11.3
Muslim	14.01	15.45	9.85	11.67	22.61	21.89	16.6	11.67
Differential	**0.08**	**-4.39**	**-2.7**	**-4.97**	**-2.82**	**-6.34**	**-3.85**	**-0.37**
Caste								
scheduled caste	20.84	13.53	7.91	9.7	24.78	17.06	13.24	12.24
Others	12.72	11.76	8.33	6.49	22.27	18.49	16.97	10.39
Differential	**8.12**	**1.77**	**-0.42**	**3.21**	**2.51**	**-1.43**	**-3.73**	**1.85**
Sector								
Rural	14.54	12.32	7.6	6.46	20.13	16.7	13.45	11.76
Urban	11.92	9.34	7.88	10.4	22.31	17.03	13.03	8.8
Differential	**2.62**	**2.98**	**-0.28**	**-3.94**	**-2.18**	**-0.33**	**0.42**	**2.96**

Source: Computed by Author from Unit Data Set of NSS 60th Round for acute and chronic ailment. And for Diarrhea and Fever the Data source used is Unit Data Set of DLHS 3.

Conclusion

The present analysis only considers outpatient care and utilisation of services yet there are number of studies documenting the fact that every year a larger number of household who are marginally above the poverty line are pushed below the poverty line on account of hospitalisation of its family members. If the poorer, rural and marginalised section of society is so prone to higher infant and child mortality, then the incidence of illness requiring hospitalisation may also be higher among them. Finally the high cost of treatment and hospitalisation may also act as a deterrent against seeking treatment, leading to prolongation of illness or even resulting in mortality in severe cases, apart from acting as a focus of infection in the community in the cases of infectious and communicable diseases.

Therefore, from the analysis made in the present chapter it is distinctly shown that there is wide disparity in treatment cost, burden of treatment, utilisation of services and consequently unequal health outcomes. There are no coherent and consistent strategies to meet the healthcare needs of the household with an equal distribution in the state of Uttar Pradesh. Assuming the further rising cost of healthcare in future particularly hospitalisation cost and the sluggishness in the economic development of these underdeveloped regions of Uttar Pradesh, we need a drastic and revolutionary change in our health policy. Any future health policy should be built on the foundation of a comprehensive establishment of primary healthcare providers for outpatient or clinical and dispensary care and comprehensive insurance plan for hospitalisation. In most of the cases it appears that actually the PHCs have failed to deliver. They are not functioning properly even if they exist at all. One major responsibility of the government is to assure access to primary healthcare to all. The present analysis has shown the urgent need for it.

Work Cited

Baru Rama, Acharya Arnab, Acharya Sanghmitra, Shiva AK, Nagraj K (2010): "Inequalities in access to Health Services in India: Caste, Class and Religion", *Economic and Political Weekly*, September 18, 2010, Vol. XLV No. 38.

Berman Peter, Ahuja Rajeev and Bhandari Laveesh (2010): "The Impoverishing Effect of Healthcare Payments in India: New Methodology and Findings", *Economic and Political Weekly*, April 17, 2010, Vol. XLV No. 16.

Dilip T.R. (2002): "Understanding Levels of Morbidity and Hospitalisation in Kerala, India", *Bulletin of the World Health Organisation* 2002, 80 (9).

Gilson, Lucy and Schneider, Helen (2007): "Understanding Health Service Access: Concepts and Experience" in Stephen Matlin in *Equitable Access: Research Challenge for Health in Developing Countries,* Global Forum Update on Research for Health Volume 4.

Gupta I (2009): "Potential Impact on Health and Economic Inequality from Cardiovascular Diseases and Diabetes in India: Evidence from the National Sample Survey", *Discussion Paper Series No. 136/2009.*

Krishnan TN (1999): "Access to Health and the Burden of Treatment in India: An Interstate Comparison", in Mohan Rao (ed.) *Disinvesting in Health: The World Bank's Prescription for Health*, Sage Publications, New Delhi, India.

Meeta and Rajivlochan (2010): "Inequalities in Health, agrarian Distress and a Policy of Avoidance", *Economic and Political Weekly*, October 23, 2010, Vol. XLV No. 43.

Peter H David, Garg Anu, Bloom Gery, Walker G Damian, Brieger R William and Rahman M Hafizpur (2008): "Poverty and access to Healthcare in Developing Countries", *New York Academy of Sciences,* 1136: 161-171.

Prabhu Seeta K (1999): "Structural Adjustment and the Health Sector in India", in Mohan Rao, *Disinvesting in Health: The World Bank's Prescription for Health,* Sage Publication, New Delhi.

Wagstaff A, Paci P, Joshi H (2001): "Causes of Inequality in Health: Who You Are? Where You Live? Or Who Your Parents Were", *Policy Research Working Paper, 2713, World Bank, Washington, DC.*

Notes

1. There are two main reasons behind taking outpatient care – one is the hospitalisation incidence occur at a very high state of illness, therefore taking hospitalisation incidences will deduct of large proportion of household bearing the burden of disease in terms of outpatient care. Moreover hospitalisation is tertiary care and its incidence is low also, therefore what is particularly important to provide basic health facility to all than to providing tertiary care to few. Indeed the Indian public health policy also focused upon providing primary healthcare to all, therefore it is more important to look at the situation here than at the tertiary level.
2. The similar kind of exercise has also been made by Krishna 1999 where he calculated the burden of treatment for various states and different deciles of population in both rural and urban area.
3. However it is hard to collect data of this as doing medical examination and collecting data is costly option on the one hand and is very tedious job on the other, required lots of human resources. Moreover if somebody is dick and needs care field investigator can't carry on collecting data leaving the person go without treatment.

Chapter 5

Public Health Expenditure and Policies in Uttar Pradesh

Health expenditure is a merit good which holds positive externalities and information asymmetries in its consumption. In the case of positive externalities and information asymmetries, the operation of market forces would alone lead to market failure or sub-optimal consumption and production of the relevant good or services, which in turn would result in an adverse impact on society's welfare (Economic Research Foundation, 2006). The available literature on effect of public health expenditure on various indicators of health outcomes and access to health services is very limited. Studies have revealed somewhat mixed result, some showing positive impact of public health expenditure upon health outcomes (Anand & Ravallion 1993; Gupta, Verhoeven and Tiongson, 1999, Bhalotra, 2006). While there are other set of studies which don't find any significant impact of public health expenditure upon health outcomes like a study done by Filmer and Pritchett (1999) on 88 developing countries shows that health expenditure has very small and statistically insignificant effect on infant and under-5 mortality. A World Bank Report (2004) reveals some of similar kind of results for the Indian states during 1980-99. However, they also show positive impact of health expenditure upon health outcomes (for child mortality) but only in the poorer states. This again has an implication that the poor states should play major role in arranging health facilities to their individual.

Using cross-sectional data for 22 developing countries in 1985, Anand and Ravallion (1993) find that health expenditure raises life expectancy and that conditional upon this, income has no effect. Similarly, using data for 50 developing and transition countries Gupta, Verhoeven and Tiongson (1999) find that health expenditure reduces childhood mortality rates. A study done by Bhalotra (2006) also explains that state health expenditure have a significant negative impact on the risk of infant mortality in India. A report by Mac Arthur Foundation (2006, p. 30) mention that improvement in a range of basic health indicators such as life expectancy at birth, infant mortality and maternal mortality can be partially traced to inadequate public expenditure and intervention. It says that there is a broad relationship with per capita health spending and some basic indicators such as life expectancy IMR and U- 5 MR. The report says that the reduced expenditure have alarming and completely adverse effect upon the health of the population, which will eventually reflect not in mortality per se but in increased morbidity and reduced capabilities.

The following correlation matrix shows that increased health expenditure holds positive impact upon the health outcomes of the masses (Table 1). It is done on the major 15 states of India for 2006 to examine the effect of public health expenditure on some selected indicators of health outcome (Death Rate, MMR, IMR, and Life Expectancy at Birth). The result shows that per capita real expenditure on health have negative association with death rate, maternal mortality rate and infant mortality rate, revealing the fact that increase in health expenditure reduces death rate, MMR and IMR. The public health expenditure explains 27 per cent variation in death rate, 18 per cent variation in MMR, 16 per cent variation in IMR. The t value for these variables are found to be greater than the tabulated value at 0.5 per cent significance level which reveals that the relative impact of per capita public health expenditure is strong. The result confirms positive association between life expectancy at birth and health expenditure, showing that 33 per cent increase in health expenditure would increase the life expectancy at birth.

Table 1

Correlation Coefficient	Correlation	r^2	T
Per Capita Revenue Expenditure on Health & Death Rate	-0.5253	0.2759	-4.715
Per Capita Revenue Expenditure on Health & MMR	-0.4255	0.1810	-3.377
Per Capita Revenue Expenditure on Health & IMR	-0.4052	0.1641	-3.151
Per Capita Revenue Expenditure on Health & Life Expectancy at Birth	0.5777	0.3337	5.635

Source: Computed by the Author.

The analysis of public health expenditure has some tribulations like government financing of health involves a number of different ministries and public sector agencies, making it difficult to arrive at entirely satisfactory estimate of government expenditure. For example, the defense institutions, railways and the number of other public organisations finance separate health systems for their employees with public funds. These are not included in accounting of public sector health spending since they are not part of the government's public health services. Besides the Ministry of Health and Family Welfare (MHFW), there are significant funding and policies are being directed by Ministry of Human Resource Development (in case of ICDS), Rural Development (Water Supply and Sanitation) etc which are not included in the health budget of government. Moreover, central, state and municipal authorities are direct financers of health service provisioning. Further government expenditure is also divided according to plan and non-plan and capital and revenue accounts and all these vary in definition and data availability. All these varied sources and varied head dealing separately having their own policies with no co-ordination with each other makes evaluation of public sector health expenditure and policies very difficult. Yet such an attempt has been made in the present chapter.

In India, the state doesn't spend even one per cent (0.90 per cent to be more specific) of GDP on health sector (Duggal, 1997; Girish, 2009), as opposed to World Health Organisation (WHO) firm stand about states spending five per cent of GDP on healthcare. As a matter of fact, of the total health expenditure in India only 15 per cent is public expenditure, the rest is private expenditure. Apparently, the investment in health sector has gone down over the years, adversely affecting healthcare of the poor and marginalised sections of the society (Girish, 2009). It needs to be noted that the share of the state governments accounts for 75 per cent of total public health expenditure. What matters more, therefore, is the financial health of the state than that of the centre. Most of the state governments suffer from acute fiscal deficit (Girish, 2009) so as the UP government also. With the present level of allocation by the state to the health sector of less than one per cent of the GDP, not even one-fourth of the health needs of the people are met. The state's lack of commitment to provide healthcare for its citizens is reflected not only in the inadequacy of the health infrastructure and low levels of financing, but also in declining people's support to the demand for public healthcare. This situation has become more pronounced since the late 1980s, coinciding with the process of liberalisation and opening up of the Indian economy to world markets.

Medical care (hospitals and dispensaries) and control of communicable diseases are crucial areas of concern both in terms of what people demand as priority areas of healthcare as well as what existing socio-economic conditions needs. As with overall public health spending, both these programmes also show declining trends in fiscal allocations in the 1980s and 1990s. In fact, in the case of disease programmes, this decline is surprising because of the large foreign assistance for AIDS and blindness control. This then means that for other crucial diseases like tuberculosis, the state's increasing disinterest in allocating resources for the health sector (family planning being an exception) is also reflected in investment expenditure; there has been a very large decline in capital expenditure during the 1990's. Further if we take into account the growth rate of inflation we would get a large negative growth for the most recent years.

The compression in health expenditure that has taken place over the last decade has resulted into altering of share of state and centre in health expenditure. It shows that the state's share in health expenditure has increased and that of central has declined drastically. Further the breakdown of central assistance to states reveals that central programmes or centrally funded programmes are of preventive in nature, which means it has serious consequences for the nation's health, especially considering that the private sector has no interest in preventive and promotive care.

Another serious problem in public health spending is the large and increasing proportion of the expenditure on salaries. This explains in part the poor use of public health services because non-salary component like medicines, fuel, equipment etc. are inadequately funded. The NIPFP database shows that commodity purchases declined steadily from 29 per cent of total expenditure in 1978 to 22 per cent in 1988 as did capital expenditure from nine per cent to seven per cent. It also reveals that real growth rate in salary expenditure during that period was 9.8 per cent and that of commodities was 5.3 per cent (Tulasidhar, 1992 *cited in* Duggal, 1997; Duggal, 2006). NCAER also found in district and municipal level study in four states that non- salary inputs ranged between 5 per cent and 21 per cent (World Bank, 1994, *cited in* Duggal, 1997). This declining share of non-salary spending will aggravate the inefficiencies within the system, further damaging the already poor status of public health services.

The major problem of health sector development in India, especially in the last two decades, has been that new programmes are begun and new facilities started with Plan funds (and an increasing amount with foreign borrowings) but their future sustenance is not completely assured by additional non-plan allocations. Health being a state subject, its sustainability is dependent on allocations made by the state. The centre has major control of plan resources and the states want to grab as large as they can. Therefore in the initial years of the plan scheme they are willing to provide matching grants, but when it is time to take charge of the programmes they shirking from their responsibilities. The programme then continues to remain a part of the plan resources with the result that new investments get affected because these old plan commitments do not get transferred to non- plan budgets. Further states have a tendency to divert programme funds away from components they are embarked for. This is largely due to the restricted role they play in policy-making and planning. This mismatch of centre state priorities have proved very expensive as funds are wasted on inadequately provided task causing allocative inefficiencies and failure of the programme to fulfil its objectives completely (Duggal, 1997).

There has been a reduction in the share of the health sector in total state government expenditure during the adjustment years, i.e. 1990-1991 to 1993-1994. The deceleration in real per capita revenue and capital expenditure on health since the mid-1980's and the decline in the share of the heath sector in total revenue expenditure in several states are bound to undermine the role of public health sector in the provisioning of health services. Over the years, with the decline in government expenditure on public health, the presence of the state in the health sector has gradually shrunk. As a result for non-hospitalised treatment, the presence of government as a service provider has shrunk from 26 per cent in 1986 to 22.3 per cent in 2003 and for urban areas, it has fallen to 19.14 per cent in 2003 from 28 per cent in 1986. For hospitalised treatment, the government sector's share has fallen from nearly 60 per cent in 1986 to 41.7 per cent in 2003. These figures cannot be taken to mean that people prefer to use the services of the private sector so far as healthcare is concerned. Private sector costs are almost three times higher as compared to cost in the public sector-Rs 8,738 for hospitalisation in the private sector as opposed to Rs 3410 in the public sector (GOUP, 2006) so for anyone with limited resources, we can safely presume, the public sector would be the default choice. However, given that public facilities are so poorly equipped, people do not have much of a choice. The NSSO (42nd round) figures show that on an average, 82 per cent in rural areas while 89 per cent in urban areas receive treatment of one kind or another. This percentage has remained fairly stable over the past 30 years. What has changed is the reason for which the remaining ill people do not take treatment. Initially the reason of not taking treatment could be traced to physical access and now to growing financial inability under increasing cost.

As the percentage of the public sector in healthcare is declining, the numbers of those who are unable to afford it are increasing. Those who either had no money or were unable to find a local medical facility were 18 per cent of all untreated morbidity in rural areas in 1986 and this figure shot up to 40 per cent by 2004. Even in urban areas, the numbers of those with no money for medical treatment doubled from 10 per cent to 20 per cent in the same period (Meeta and Rajivlochan, 2010).

In post-independence India what initially started as a programme for eradicating malaria and small pox resulted into a huge infrastructure of public health in the 1950s and 1960s. During the 1960s and 1970s primary level health services grew, largely due to the pumping of funds for the vertical single disease control programmes and the family planning programmes. With too much emphasis on family planning, the PHCs lost orientation and curative health delivery services were neglected. Call it sluggishness or the sheer inability of the states to check these programmes, the downslide further escalated in the 1980's leading to a spurt in the private sector. The mounting fiscal crisis in the country turned out to be the fatal blow given such a dismal condition. Thus, what necessitated health sector reforms was essentially a cumulative effect of a series of unfavourable developments coupled with misguided perception of the appropriate use of health sector infrastructure as well as the inability of the state to confront with the problems emanating from several sources plus fiscal crisis. Needless to say, the 1991 economic reforms had already cleared the deck for the stated purpose. However, with the unfolding of health sector reforms, there has been a paradigm shift wherein the conceptualisation of healthcare has changed from a service to a commodity (for which everybody has to pay) (Girish, 2009).

Besides the amount of expenditure another major problem is its miss-allocation due to guidelines from varied sources which at times resulted into extra focus to certain areas with a little focus to the area requiring attention. For instance in case of the programme of Family Planning in UP during 1998-99 to 2002-03 the expenditure on FW increased by 12.30 per cent with a negative increase of 1.47 per cent on Medical and Public Health in the same period. It has also been criticised that FW programmes are not cost-effective and they are taking a bulk of money with very little impact on health of the population. Moreover in UP a kind of biasedness in public health expenditure can be seen for urban areas, preventive care and primary health sector. It has resulted into greater disparity in disease burden on rural people and rising health cost due to lack of health facility at secondary and tertiary level. Negligence of preventive health system resulted into outburst of disease, say for example the spread of Japanese Encephalitis in Tarai region of Uttar Pradesh take a great toll of money and lives and increases the burden upon curative care. Thus, a kind of miss-match between health policy and expenditure can be visualised looking at the minor heads of the budget of state.

The above discussion makes the point that low per capita public health expenditure in states with larger concentration of poverty results into high out of pocket expenditure which is highly regressive in nature and leads to low access to health services particularly for poor. In Uttar Pradesh the scarcity of formal public services forces the people to go to private practitioners, local experts or quacks or to go without proper treatment. Thus, given the above discussion the present chapter examines the trend of public healthcare expenditure in Uttar Pradesh, its impact upon health infrastructure and health outcome. While doing so the chapter also analyses the public health expenditure in the state in combination with policy shifts at state as well as centres level and how they have affected each other. Finally the chapter concludes with an explanation of health sector condition of Uttar Pradesh in consequence of public healthcare policies and public health expenditure.

I. Basic Characteristics of Health Expenditure in Uttar Pradesh

Health spending in Uttar Pradesh is very low at 1.4 per cent of GSDP in 2007-08. This expenditure is sum total of revenue and capital expenditure on medicine and public health, family welfare, expenditure on water and sanitation and nutrition. As a consequence most of the burden is born by out of pocket expenditure of the individual, and a scenario of more than one-third of population below poverty line renders great many people to suffer from preventable mortality and premature deaths. Given the imperatives the low level of public expenditure has generated drawing out effect and created space for private sector to flourish and the market resources to play independently. Low level of public spending has particularly resulted into poor infrastructure for preventive healthcare (Rao and Choudhary) as well as shortage of health centres and health personals (Table 4). Thus, the poor state of health infrastructure has forced the less privileged to seek care from unregulated high cost private health providers, with huge adverse effects. Consequently it has resulted into poor health outcomes and access to health services in the state. The immunisation rate against various diseases like measles, tuberculosis etc is very low (*cf* Chapter 2). Same is the case with access to various healthcare services like population coverage to clean water supply, contraceptive use, births attended by skilled personnel and the ratio of physicians to total population (*cf* Chapter 2).

Healthcare in UP is primarily financed by private spending with out of pocket expenditure accounting for over 71 per cent of the total expenditure. The total non-public sector spending on heath accounts for 83 per cent and government healthcare funding accounts for mere 17 per cent to the total spending (GOUP, 2006). Moreover average medical expenditure per hospitalisation case in rural UP in the public sector is estimated at Rs 7648. This is more than twice as much as the national average of Rs 3238. This does not include loss of household income. Even the cost in the private sector is found to be much higher in UP than the national average. In the urban areas too, the cost of healthcare in the public sector is much higher in UP than the national average (GOUP, 2006).

National Health Accounts (2005) estimates indicate that the household sector spends Rs 17158 crore on health in UP whereas government spends only Rs 2650 crore. In Kerala, the household sector spends only Rs 8373 crore, while in Tamil Nadu household sector spends Rs 3624 crore only. This makes it amply clear that it is not so much the shortage of resources as it is the inappropriate organisation and flow of resources. Much of the out of pocket expenses comes from the pockets of ordinary citizens. They spend through their assets, often falling into poverty and ends up getting inappropriate care (GOUP, 2006).

II. Trends in Health Expenditure in Uttar Pradesh

Health is a state subject and therefore financing is primarily by the state governments. Resource allocation to this sector is influenced by the general fiscal situation of the state government. For instance, the implementation of the recommendations of the Fifth Pay Commission during the late 1990s resulted in an increase in the fiscal deficit and a general resource crunch (MOHFW, 2005). At the very time when reforms measures were initiated at the Centre during the early 1990s, fiscal transfers to states were compressed leading to reductions in health sector allocation. By the year 2001-02, the relative allocation to the sector reached levels closer to those prevailing in 1975-76 (MOHFW, 2005). Moreover the allocation of health resources by the centre favours the richer states. Therefore instead of allocating fund on the basis of the individual need of the states, some of communicable disease programmes are funded on a fifty-fifty basis by the state and central budget (MOHFW, 2005) which mainly centred to richer state. The conclusion of above discussion is that at one hand UP is expending low on health services due to poor economic resources and on the other hand centre's assistance to health have been very low. The diagram (Figure 1 and Figure 2) given below is an analysis of public health expenditure as percentage of GSDP and real per capita public health expenditure of Kerala and UP from 1987-88 to 2007-08. It reveals that the public health expenditure as percentage of GSDP in Uttar Pradesh has been very low than the public health expenditure by Kerala from early 1987. It has shown an improvement only after 2003-04 and from there onwards it is more than Kerala's health expenditure. Still, the real per capita public expenditure on health in Uttar Pradesh is far below the real per capita public health expenditure of Kerala. But earlier neglect of health sector in UP can't be offset by the later increase in public health expenditure. Moreover, that increase is too low to achieve the health goals.

Moreover, the public health expenditure as percentage of GSDP has shown very low level of increasing trend in UP, but it does not show such trend in terms of real per capita health expenditure. Given the increasing growth of population in the state and poor health status of the masses due to initial negligence of health sector in Uttar Pradesh, it demands greater attention to health sector in fund allocation. However, after 2005 Uttar Pradesh being a high focused state has received larger fund under the NRHM programme but it is yet to produce effective outcomes.

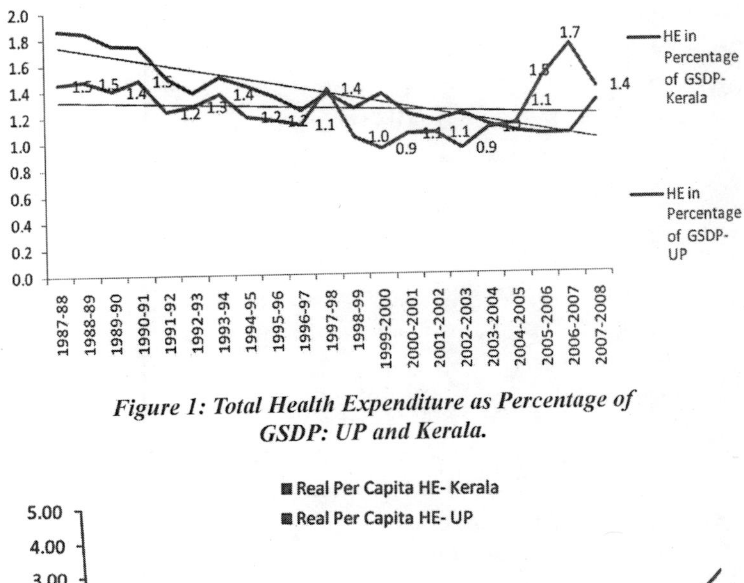

Figure 1: Total Health Expenditure as Percentage of GSDP: UP and Kerala.

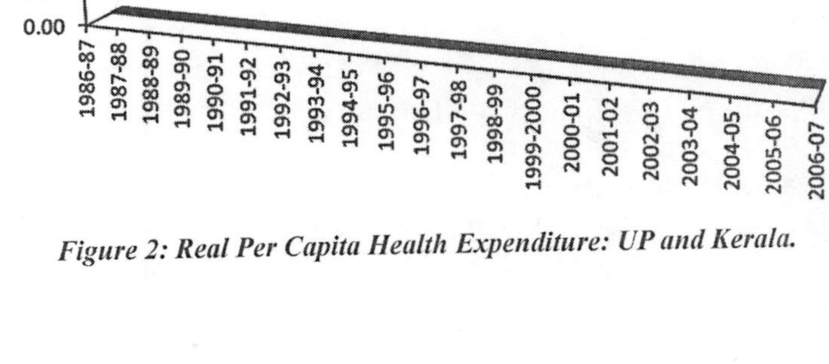

Figure 2: Real Per Capita Health Expenditure: UP and Kerala.

Many important trends in the public health expenditure of the state are discernable. The state is required to expend on the policy formulated by the centre and the latter did not pay attention to the state specific priorities. As a result following Bhore committee report, health and family welfare became the policy priority of the UP and other states also. It has allocated about 3.3 per cent of national plan expenditures in the first five year plan, with a negligence of general medicine and preventive care. In subsequent years, at national level public investment strategy gave greater priority to economic growth and industrialisation with resultant reductions in health spending as a proportion of the total. During this period states health expenditure also decreased due to shrinkage of funding from centre and state's emphasis on GDP growth. Another shock to public health expenditure has been SAP (Structural Adjustment Programme) and the situation further got deteriorated as a consequence of the fifth pay commission implementation around 1996 – 98. It has shrink the non-salary components in the public health expenditure (Duggal, 2005). Thus, a greater reliance on the market for healthcare access becomes more difficult for increasing number of people. The evidence of galloping out of pocket expenditure and indebtedness for supporting healthcare expenditure is reflected from NSS 42nd and 52nd rounds, where utilisation of health services has substantially increased and being funded by the borrowings of the households.

However, this trend has been largely reversed in sixth and seventh plans with health and water sanitation each now exceeding 3.5 per cent of plan allocations at central level. In Uttar Pradesh also during the same period expenditure increased upon water and sanitation with less attention to general medicine and public health.

During this period the increase in health expenditure of the state of Uttar Pradesh is largely due to growing importance of central government financed and co-financed schemes such as the family welfare programme, the rural water supply programme and most recently the universal immunisation programme within FW (Table 2). In general in Uttar Pradesh the budgetary head of FW showed much greater variation across the sub-periods than the other category. But the most dramatic decline in per capita spending is on Medical and PH. The lack of life saving medical equipment in the hospitals is a great reflection of this.

Table 2: Annual Rates of Growth of Expenditure by Category: UP & Kerala

Kerala	*1993-94-1997-98*	*1998-99- 2002-03*
Medical and Public Health	2.42	4.71
FW	-2.99	-0.62
Uttar Pradesh		
Medical and Public Health	4.24	-1.47
FW	-0.45	12.30

Source: Mac Arthur Foundation, 2006.

The increments in public health expenditures, especially through centrally-supported schemes, have been marked by increasing emphasis on rural services and primary healthcare, including continued investment in lower level rural health facilities and personnel and community level service schemes. Meanwhile the government of UP also started placing importance on primary healthcare. Consequently, there has been too much of focus on primary health with the neglect of secondary and tertiary health (Table 3).

Table 3: Sectoral Allocation of Health Expenditure by States: 2001- 02

States	*Primary (Lakhs)*	*Secon-dary (Lakhs)*	*Tertiary (Lakhs)*	*Soc. Health Ins. lakhs)*	*Adminis-trative (Lakhs)*	*Res.& Trg. (Lakhs)*
Well Performing States						
Andhra Pradesh	63241	22844	27625	5419	11592	2326
	-47.53	-17.17	-20.76	-4.07	-8.71	-1.75
Karnataka	51334	23883	23626	4719	4164	844
	-47.28	-22	-21.76	-4.35	-3.83	-0.78
Kerala	19389	26460	21198	3502	1979	2385
	-25.88	-35.32	-28.3	-4.67	-2.64	-3.18
Tamil Nadu	52700	18120	34114	8011	5266	1772
	-43.92	-15.1	-28.43	-6.68	-4.39	-1.48

(Contd...)

Medium Performing States						
Punjab	26078	10078	9419	3131	12140	995
	-42.17	-16.3	-15.23	-5.06	-19.63	-1.61
Gujarat	30336	4986	20430	6623	8968	1558
	-41.61	-6.84	-28.02	-9.09	-12.3	-2.14
Haryana	16217	5060	5507	2436	2518	412
	-50.38	-15.72	-17.11	-7.57	-7.82	-1.28
West Bengal	46184	35376	30153	6737	12457	1839
	-34.79	-26.65	-22.71	-5.07	-9.38	-1.39
Maharashtra	102106	27722	36292	11120	4645	1380
	-55.7	-15.12	-19.8	-6.07	-2.53	-0.75
Poor Performing States						
Assam	21002	6003	6109	0	2182	314
	-58.98	-16.86	-17.16	0	-6.13	-0.88
Bihar	46349	6047	11728	768	4765	1692
	-64.96	-8.48	-16.44	-1.08	-6.68	-2.37
Madhya Pradesh	41650	10791	14420	2049	4915	1771
	-54.14	-14.03	-18.74	-2.66	-6.39	-2.3
Orissa	20370	11837	6590	1054	4407	645
	-45.33	-26.34	-14.66	-2.34	-9.81	-1.43
Rajasthan	57831	7556	24598	2275	5159	1419
	-58.5	-7.64	-24.88	-2.3	-5.22	-1.44
Uttar Pradesh	142193	50257	18138	6680	12034	621
	-61.18	-21.62	-7.8	-2.87	-5.18	-0.27
Total	**754143**	**269369**	**291486**	**64850**	**98346**	**20366**
	-50.18	**-17.92**	**-19.4**	**-4.32**	**-6.54**	**-1.36**

Source: Report on Macro Economics and Health.

Table 3 suggest that an equitable spread of resources among all the three sectors-primary, secondary and tertiary is necessary. As can be seen in the case of UP, the skewed spending on primary and negligible amount on tertiary sector, which deals with medical colleges and training, can have long-term effectson the quality of people trained or in creating a shortage of skilled personnel. Whether inadequate in number or poorly trained, the impact on access to primary care services will be adverse, as the care provided will ultimately depend on the human resources available (MHFW & WHO, 2005). Moreover, the major share of the resources has gone to curative services, as of 1990-91, a little more than 60 per cent of the resources had gone to curative services, 26 per cent to preventive services and the remaining percentage to administration and miscellaneous services. This reflects the misallocation of resources in Uttar Pradesh despite moderate increase in health expenditure. Another important point is that real per capita expenditure in UP is far below Kerala. Although the expenditure as percentage of GSDP has increased in recent times but it has failed to compensate for the ever rising population of the state.

Further, the average healthcare expenditure in rural areas is very low (33 per cent) in comparison to urban areas (66 per cent). Thus, the relationship between share of resources devoted to rural health sector and the share of rural population may not be in line with objective of achieving health for all (Bansal, 1999). Further the public curative and hospital services are mostly in cities while in rural areas there are only preventive and promotive services like FP and immunisation. As a result private sector plays a very important role in health delivery system of rural area especially under-qualified persons and quacks (Duggal, 2005). In response to this government has started altogether rural centric new initiative through National Rural Health Mission in 2005. This primarily focuses on developing primary level health services mainly for maternal and child health at village level.

The period after 1983 witnessed several major developments in the polices impacting the health sector - adoption of National Health Policy in 1983, 73rd and 74th Constitutional Amendments in 1992, National Nutrition Policy in 1993, National Health Policy in 2002, National Policy on Indian System of Medicine and Homeopathy in 2002, Drug Policy in 2002, introduction of Universal Health Insurance Schemes for the Poor in 2003 and inclusion of health in Common Minimum Programme of the UPA Government in 2004. The first National Health Policy in 1983 aimed to achieve the goal of 'Health for All' by 2000 AD, through the provision of comprehensive primary healthcare services. It stressed the creation of an infrastructure for primary healthcare; close co-ordination with health-related services and activities (like nutrition, drinking water supply and sanitation); the active involvement and participation of voluntary organisations; the provision of essential drugs and vaccines; qualitative improvement in health and family planning services; the provision of adequate training; and medical research aimed at the common health problems of the people.

Through the 73rd (1993) and 74th (1994) Constitutional Amendment Acts the local bodies (Panchayat and Municipalities) have been assigned 29 and 18 development activities respectively. The transfer of functions include health and sanitation (covering hospitals, PHCs and dispensaries), family welfare, drinking water, women and child development, the public distribution system and poverty alleviation programmes.

The Common Minimum Programme announced by the UPA government in 2004 has proposed to raise public spending on health to at least 2-3 per cent of the Gross Domestic Product (GDP) over the next five years with focus on primary healthcare. The present government has proposed to take all steps to ensure availability of life saving drugs at reasonable prices through revival of public sector units in the manufacture of critical bulk drugs.

The main objective of the revised National Health Policy, 2002 is to achieve an acceptable standard of good health among the general population of the country and has set goals to be achieved by the year 2015. The major policy implications are as follows:

- Increase public expenditure from 0.9 per cent to two per cent by 2010.
- Increase allocation of public health investment in the order of 55 per cent for the primary health sector; 35 per cent and 10 per cent to secondary and tertiary sectors respectively.
- Gradual convergence of all health programmes, except the ones (such as TB, Malaria, HIV/AIDS, RCH), which need to be continued till moderate levels of prevalence are reached.
- Need to levy user charges for certain secondary and tertiary public health services, for those who can afford to pay.
- Mandatory two-year rural posting before awarding the graduate medical degree.

- Decentralising the implementation of health programmes to local self-governing bodies by 2005.
- Setting up of Medical Grants Commission for funding new Government Medical and Dental colleges.
- Establishing two-tier urban healthcare system - Primary Health Centre for a population of one lakh and Government General Hospital.
- Increase in Government funded health research to a level of two per cent of the total health spending by 2010.
- Appreciation of the role of private sector in health, and enactment of legislation by 2003 for regulating private clinical establishments.
- Formulation of procedures for accreditation of public and private health facilities.
- Full operationalisation of National Disease Surveillance Network by 2005.
- Notification of contemporary code of medical ethics by Medical Council of India.
- Encouraging setting up of private insurance instruments to bring secondary and tertiary sectors into its purview.
- Encouragement and promotion of Indian System of Medicine.

III. Consequences of Compression in Health Expenditure

A comparison of public health expenditure as percentage of GSDP of Kerala and UP from 1987-88 to 2007-08 reveals that it has been very low in UP. right from 1987. It has shown an improvement only after 2003-04 and from there onwards it is closer to Kerala's health expenditure. But earlier neglect of health sector in UP can't be compensated by the latter increase in public health expenditure. Moreover, that increase is too low to achieve the health goals. The real per capita public expenditure on health in Uttar Pradesh is far below the real per capita public health expenditure of Kerala. That means a small increase in absolute expenditure has been offset by the increased population and could not make any effective impact. As a consequence it has generated a huge shortfall in the public health sector of UP in terms of physical as well as personnel. In comparison to major fifteen states UP stands almost at the top in terms of shortfall in all the indicators of health infrastructure and human resources; be it specialist male and female workers, PHCs, CHCs or Sub-centres (Table 4).

Table 4: Shortfall in Personnel and Physical Infrastructure in Health Sector of UP vis-a-vis. India and States

	Personnel Shortfall				*Shortfall in Physical Infrastructure*			
	Specialist	*Male Worker*	*Female Worker*	*Average*	*Sub Centres*	*PHCs*	*CHCs*	*Average*
Andhra Pradesh	75.15	51.07	14.85	47.02	0	18.41	65.28	27.90
Assam	N/A	N/A	*	N/A	*	26.15	51.46	38.80
Bihar	62.86	86.08	15.66	54.87	40.44	33.79	83.92	52.72
Haryana	88.66	82.53	32.88	68.02	19.45	17.8	31.2	22.82
Kerala	73.13	16.25	6.15	31.85	0	0	45.69	15.23
Madhya Pradesh	53.43	25.74	13.95	31.04	15.07	31.20	35.25	27.17
Maharashtra	72.48	41.67	21.67	45.27	13.99	9.27	17.94	13.74
Orissa	N/A	42.77	6.08	24.43	18.62	*	20.89	19.75
Punjab	64.88	51.89	24.75	47.17	11.21	9.70	5.97	8.96
Rajasthan	55.49	76.18	*	65.83	*	*	13.14	13.14
Tamil Nadu	23.20	82.69	*	52.94	0	0	19.45	6.48
West Bengal	54.91	50.00	12.22	39.04	14.42	53.74	30.52	32.89
Uttar Pradesh	73.25	72.07	9.43	51.58	22.10	16.63	75.23	37.99
Rank of UP	3	5	8	5	2	7	1	2
India	**58.44**	**56.71**	**12.62**	**42.59**	**13.13**	**18.57**	**38.90**	**23.54**

Source: Health Information of India, 2005,*- Surplus, N/A- Data Not Available.

Moreover the mismatched policies have also resulted into poor access and health outcomes of the masses in UP. Like the dramatic decline in per capita spending on Medical and PH has resulted into lack of life saving medical equipment in the hospitals and inadequacies in various other requirements. In UP the expenditure on medical and public health has seen negative growth rate of -1.47 per cent during the time period of 1998-2002 as opposed to 12.30 per cent increase in the expenditure on Family Welfare during the same time period. It has generated a scenario where all the resources of public health centres have been mobilised for the schemes of family welfare programme (Table 2). The programmes of Family Welfare have become the policy priority at national level. In the first five year plan it has been allocated about 3.3 per cent of national plan expenditures as part of World Bank project for population control. It has been more forcefully implemented in UP as it is the most populous state facing highest growth rate of population. The altogether lower allocation of funding to health sector created low funding to general medicine and preventive care and as a result negligence of these sector. A study (Duggal, 2006) reveals a very alarming fact that in 1990's there have been improvements in primary health centres but the mobilisation of resources for FW converted these centres as instrument for population control and thereby missing their primary priority of ensuring primary healthcare services to all.

The small amount of expenditure on health sector combined with mismatched policies has resulted into a situation where burden of health expenditure on the budget of household has increased dramatically. Several rounds of NSS and various studies keep on reporting that a substantial amount of expenditure of household is going to finance health expenditure. In UP, 71 per cent health expenditure is born by the household and only 17 per cent comes from the public sector. It has created a huge burden on the pocket of individual where the rich and better off can bear it given their purchasing power but the poor and marginalised has to go without health services.

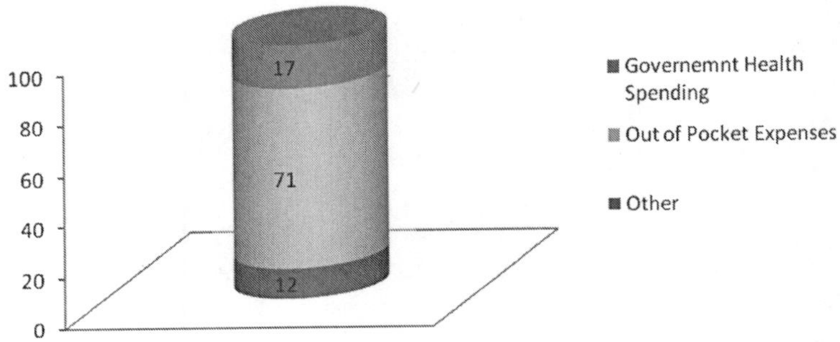

Figure 3: Proportion of Private and Public Spending on Health in Uttar Pradesh – 2004-05.

As can be seen by the table given below that in UP loss of income because of medical expenditure is huge and well above the national average. However the condition is worse in rural areas where the loss of income due to the health expenditure is almost double the loss of income in urban areas (Table 5).

Table 5: Average Medical Expenditure Per 000 Hospitalisation Case in Rural and Urban UP and India

	Rural			*Urban*		
	Public	*Loss of Private*	*Income*	*Public*	*Private*	*Loss of Income*
UP	7648	9169	920	5144	10351	536
India	3238	7408	636	3877	11553	745

GOUP, 2006.

Therefore given such a gloomy condition of health sector of UP, facing huge shortfall in its health infrastructure and health personnel, increasing cost of health services are bound to negatively affect the health of the masses. As is evident from the Table 6 given below UP is one of the high focused states in NRHM scheme. A very important scheme started in 2005 to improve the health of the worst performing states in particular and of all states in general.

IV. Which section of population is the most affected by such compression

In order to get the answer of this research question we have to first look at who are the worst sufferers in terms of health outcomes and then who are going to avail health facilities from the public providers. If these two groups are same then it is evidently concluded that it is this particular section who is the worst affected by contraction in public health expenditure.

First looking at the health outcomes of the people from various socio-economic groups reveals that in all categories of mortality indicators urban UP is better than rural UP (Table 7). All mortality rates are always higher in rural area and Hindu religious group. A child of a SC mother has lower chance of survival than any other

Table 6: Key Demographic Indicators

States	*Per capita Expenditure*	*Life Expectancy at Birth (2002-06)*	*IMR 2008*	*MMR - 2008*	*TFR 2008-09*	*Any Anemia-Men*	*Any Anemia-Women*	*Full Immunisation*	*% Safe Delivery*
High Focus EAG States									
Bihar	513	61.6	56	312	3.9	34.3	67.4	32.8	18
Madhya Pradesh	789	58	70	335	3.3	25.6	56	40.3	32
Orissa	902	59.6	69	303	2.4	33.9	61.2	51.8	37
Rajasthan	761	62	63	388	3.3	23.6	53.1	26.5	38
Uttar Pradesh	974	60	67	440	3.8	24.3	49.9	23	26
General Category States									
Andhra Pradesh	1061	64.4	52	154	1.8	23.3	62.9	46	68
Gujarat	953	64.1	50	160	2.5	22.2	55.3	45.2	60
Haryana	1078	66.2	54	186	2.5	19.2	56.1	65.3	44
Karnataka	830	65.3	45	213	2	19.1	51.5	55	62
Kerala	2950	74	12	95	1.7	8	32.8	75.3	97
Maharashtra	1212	67.2	33	130	2	16.8	48.4	58.8	61
Punjab	1359	69.4	41	192	1.9	13.6	38	60.1	61
Tamil Nadu	1256	66.2	31	111	1.7	16.5	53.2	80.9	80
West Bengal	1259	64.9	35	141	1.9	32.3	63.2	64.3	43
INDIA	**1201**	**63.5**	**53**	**254**	**2.6**	**24.2**	**55.3**	**43.5**	-

Source: Facility Survey. DLHS- 3- 2007-08.

caste groups. Wealth appears to improve child survival chances across all mortality rates. Therefore, it is the poor and marginalised facing highest mortality rate. Obviously these groups must be facing highest burden of ailment and as a result are in greater need of accessing public healthcare facilities at affordable price. In fact it is this group who are facing highest burden of treatment in all regions of UP.

Table 7: Some Important Indicators of Child Health by Characteristics

Background Characteristics	*Neonatal Mortality*	*Postnatal Mortality*	*Infant Mortality*	*Child Mortality*	*Under 5 Mortality*
Residence					
Urban	43.8	28.4	72.7	24.3	94.8
Rural	57.7	28.1	85.8	34	116.9
Religion					
Hindu	57.2	28	85.2	33.5	115.8
Muslim	46.9	29.7	76.5	26.6	101.1
Social Group					
SCs	60.2	30.5	90.7	48.9	135.1
OBCs	58.9	25.2	84.1	29.4	111
Other	38.1	33.3	71.4	17.6	87.7
Wealth Quintiles					
Lowest	65.3	28.9	94.2	45.5	135.4
Second	54.7	30.1	84.8	35.3	117.1
Middle	57	32.7	89.7	27.7	114.9
Fourth	43	24.7	67.7	17.5	84
Highest	35.2	16.2	51.3	11.1	61.8
Total	**54.8**	**28.2**	**83**	**32**	**112.3**

Source: NFHS- 3, 2006.

Further, it has been made clear while discussing utilisation of public health services in Chapter - 5 that it is the poor and marginalised group of the society who are going to seek treatment from public providers for their health needs. (Chapter 4, Section 3, Table 6). Consequently, the poor and people from lower strata of society are the worst affected by such compression in public health expenditure. Because the rich and better off section of the society can go to private providers with their higher purchasing power, better negotiation capacity and social networks.

Thus, it is clear from above discussion that poor and marginalised people are the most likely to be ill and they are largely relying on public providers for their health needs. Therefore, it is this section which is affected by the shrinking of public healthcare expenditure and there by shrinking government role in provisioning of healthcare needs of the population. In fact there is already a very clear case of this section, largely dying in silence with a combination of highest mortality rate and lowest reporting of diseases. Therefore, if government further reduces its role in health sector, it is bound to affect the health of the poor and marginalised.

Moreover empirical evidences concerning the impact of public spending on the health status of countries' population have also found that the poor are significantly less healthy than the rich and it is those who are less likely to obtain care when sick. Moreover, in the case if poor obtain healthcare, it is from public provided facilities. These suggest the public spending on health matter more for the individual from lower socio-economic status (SES)[1] because they rely more on public health resources while non-poor are able to substitute private spending for public spending (Gupta, Verhoeven and Tiongson, 2002; Bidani and Ravallion 1997). These studies also support the conclusion drawn above. However, there are very few studies which have assessed the impact of public health expenditure on poor's health outcome. A study done by World Bank (1995) on Philippines also came up with similar kind of result. One more study done by Deolalikar (1995) on Indonesia also finds that the marginal impact of public health spending on the incidence and duration of children's illness is slightly larger on the poor than the non-poor.

Conclusion

Through all this discussion it is clear that the resources available are insufficient to meet everyone's needs on equitable basis. Though the Bhore commission recommended for large increase in public health spending, but there has not been sufficient rise in public health expenditure, largely because health has not been the policy priority of central and in the present context of UP government. In this case Kerala is a classic example which has always accorded high priority to health. The Kerala government has made more focused and coordinated attempts in health sector which made it ideal state in India as well as globally in terms of social sector achievement.

Moreover, the misallocation of resources has been a major problem in public health expenditure, larger amount of the medical and public health goes to paying salaries of the staff and the expenditure on drugs is neglected. Since long the expenditure on revenue account is increasing but expenditure on capital account is not following the same trend and as a result the new equipments (oxygen cylinder, bed, pathology) new buildings, ambulance and other assets are not created in health centres. This is quite evident by the DLHS facility survey that in UP more than 70 per cent public institutions are not well equipped. Lack of these basic resources makes people seek care from private health providers. A very meagre amount of expenditure goes to rural area where bulk of people lived. Even that too did not generate secondary and tertiary health centres and as a result there is widening inequality in health outcome of urban and rural people. Further the state has neglected the precaution is better than cure policy and focused its expenditure on curative care as a result at times outburst of disease occurred, which could have been prevented if state has taken prior notice of that. It means that increased attention to preventive care is more important than that of curative care oriented health policy. Therefore, the lack of resources is one and the misallocation of the small resources has been the other major problem in the whole public health expenditure system of the state of Uttar Pradesh. These two things affected the health outcomes of the people of state very badly.

However, Health expenditure is not the sole determinant of health outcomes. Given wide expenditure on health there are certain other dimensions which have adverse impact upon health outcomes. Most importantly evidences on poor health outcomes suggest "underutilisation of health services and infrastructure to be critical in hampering the expected influence of public expenditure on improving health outcomes. This underutilisation is sometimes interpreted as indicating a low level of demand for social services.

However, Minhas (1991) has explained the under utilisation in education reflecting supply side constraints, particularly the poor quality of services provided in most publicly funded institution. Prabhu (2001) also has shown that the impact of government expenditure on social attainment depends critically on the efficiency of the functioning of delivery system. Some other factors like corruption, absenteeism by the health personnel and bad treatment at the health centres are also important reasons for poor access to health services and consequently to bad health outcomes. The present discussion shows that merely expenditure on health is not the guarantee of improvement in health outcomes rather concerted effort by the state is the pre-requisite.

Work Cited

Anand S and Ravallion M (1993): "Human Development in Poor Countries: On the Role of Private Incomes and Public Services", *Journal of Economic Perspectives,* 1 (3).

Bansal RD (1999): "Health Financing in India: Priorities, Issues, Inter-State Variations and Challenges", *Health and Population- Perspectives and Issues* 22 (3&4): 123-132.

Berman P (1991): "Health Economics, Health Financing and the Health Needs of Poor Women and Children in India", *The Ford Foundation,* New Delhi.

Berman P, Ahuja R and Bhandari L (2010): "The Impoverishing Effect of Healthcare Payments in India: New Methodology and Findings", *Economic and Political Weekly,* April 17, 2010, Vol, XLV No. 16.

Bhalotra S: "Spending to Save? State Health Expenditure and Infant Mortality in India", *Department of Economics and CMPO, University of Bristol.*

Bidani B and Ravallion M (1997): "Decomposing Social Indicators Using Distributional Data", *Journal of Econometrics,* 77: 125- 139.

Deolalikar AB (1995): "Government Health Spending in Indonesia: Impact on Children in Different Economic Groups" in Walle D and Nead K, *Public Spending and the Poor: Theory and Evidence,* Johns Hopkins University Press: Baltimore.

Duggal Ravi (2005): "Public Health Expenditures, Investment and Financing Under the Shadow of a Growing Private Sector", in Gangolli V Leena, Duggal R and Shukla Abhay, *Review of Health Care in India,* Center for Equity into Health and Allied Themes (CEHAT).

——— (2006): "Utilisation of Health Care Services in India" in Prasad Sujata and Sathyamala C, *Securing Health For All: Dimensions and Challenges,* Institute for Human Development, New Delhi.

Filmer D and Pritchett L (1999): "The Impact of Public Spending on Health: Does Money Matter?" *Social Science and Medicine,* 49 (10), 1309-1323.

Government of Uttar Pradesh (2006): "Human Development Report of Uttar Pradesh".

Government of India (2005): "Health Statistics of India", Ministry of Health and Family Welfare, Government of India.

Gupta S, Verhoeven M and Tiongson E (1999): "Does Higher Government Spending Buy Better Results in Education and Health Care?" *Washington DC: International Monetary Fund,* Working Paper 99/21.

IIPS and Macro International (2007): "National and Family Health Survey-3", 2005-06: India: VL, 1. Mumbai, IIPS.

IIPS and WHO (2006): "World Health Survey, 2003- India", International Institute for Population Sciences (IIPS), Mumbai, World Health Organisation, Geneva, World Health Organisation- India- WR Office, New Delhi.

MacArthur Foundation (2006): "Government Health Expenditure in India: A Benchmark Study", *Economic Research Foundation,* New Delhi.

Minhas BS (1991): "Educational Deprivation and its Role as a Spoiler of Access to Better Life in India", *Indian Statistical Institute,* Technical Report No. 9104, Kolkata.

Ministry of Health and Family Welfare (2005): "Report of the National Commission on Macroeconomics and Health", Government of India.

———— (2007- 08): "District Level Household and Facility Survey under Reproductive and Child Health Project (DLHS-3)", International Institute of Population Sciences, Mumbai.

NIPFP (2005): "Health Care Status in India", National Institute of Public Finance and Policy, New Delhi.

Prabhu K Seeta (2001): *Economic Reform and Social Sector Development: A Study of Two Indian States*, United Nations Development Programme, New Delhi, Sage Publications, New Delhi.

Rao Govind M and Choudgary Mita: "Inter State Equalisation of Health Expenditure in Indian Union", *National Institute of Public Finance and Policy*, New Delhi.

World Bank, Philippines (1995): "Public Expenditure Management for Sustained and Equitable growth", *World Bank Report* No. 14680- PH, Washington.

Notes

1. The literature on socio-economic inequality in health examine the distribution of health by occupational class, educational attainment, income, dwelling size, consumption and ownership of certain asset i.e. wealth index. For the present work we have taken religion, social group, residential characteristics, consumption expenditure to examine SES in the distribution of health.

Chapter 6

Conclusion

This study explores the scale and magnitude of unjust and unfair access or non-access to public healthcare services and health outcomes in state of Uttar Pradesh, primarily using secondary data sources like NFHS-3, DLHS-3 and NSS- 60th round. Therefore, the present study is an attempt to explore the role of public resources in determining the access to healthcare services i.e. accessibility, affordability, utilisation and acceptability of healthcare services in various regions of Uttar Pradesh and among socio-economic group.

The analysis and interpretation carried out so far reveals that Uttar Pradesh is a state having severe shortage of health personal and health infrastructure. Variations in the availability of public health services can be seen in terms of requisites infrastructure, human resources, appropriate medical equipments and health institutions among the various regions of the Uttar Pradesh. "It is a matter of contemporary fact that health facility in India have collapsed. Public health facilities are close to non-existent and private health services far too few, far too exploitative and focused mainly on the urban areas" (Meeta and Rajivlochan, 2010, p. 41).

In terms of availability of public health institutions (any government health facility) Bundelkhand region is having highest percentages of villages i.e. 47.97 per cent where any government health facility is available followed by central, eastern and then western region. Indeed it shows a very alarming condition in terms of average population coverage too. In all regions there is huge population pressure on the sub-centres, CHCs and PHCs and one can imagine the population pressure on tertiary healthcare facility given the fact that there is only one public hospital in a district to provide the referral care to rural as well as urban population. However, what is particularly important is to have the health personnel in these centres to provide any treatment or medicine. It is shown that most of them are not well equipped. In this respect it is western UP which is doing better than the state average. In terms of the availability of doctors 31.37 per cent villages are having doctors in western UP as opposed to mere 9.64 per cent in central and 14.27 per cent in eastern regions. Similarly, 93.3 per cent villages have Anganwadi worker in western UP, well above other regions and state average. Western UP is having 74.11 per cent 24 hour functioning PHCs as against only 30.4 per cent in eastern UP and 85.28 per cent PHCs having at least four beds as against just half in eastern region.

Affordability of healthcare services incorporates the direct and indirect cost of treatment and households capacity to meet those costs (Gilson *et al,* 2007; Baru *et al*, 2010). Affordability in combination with public health provisioning determines equal/ unequal access to healthcare services and health outcome. The public healthcare provisioning definitely reduces cost of healthcare and improves access of economically poor.

Adverse socio-economic differential in average total expenditure is a situation wide spread in all regions of UP, but the situation is the worst in Bundelkhand. The regional variation in socio-economic differential in health expenditure is shown from the fact that the average expenditure on health is very low among the Muslims than Hindu. The gap is especially higher in eastern UP (183.76) followed by Bundelkhand (169.41). Similar is the case in caste groups. Here the gap in average expenditure is higher in central UP followed by Bundelkhand. In terms of economic groups and rural-urban residence inequality is the highest in Bundelkhand. However, it is worth mentioning here that from the low expenditure on health one should not infer the lack of disease in any particular group. Rather it means that the group is not seeking health services. It may be a case of either deliberate under reporting or ignorance about the disease itself. Given the fact that burden of communicable and chronic diseases are continuously increasing and findings from NSS 50, 55th and 61st rounds of households consumption expenditure reporting continuous rise in share of medical expenditure in households total consumption expenditure, it definitely cannot be interpreted as lack of disease.

Based on the analysis of data from the NSS - 60th round it is shown that the high burden of expenditure on healthcare is largely financed through two major sources, namely, households own resources and borrowings. Borrowing is one of the important sources of health expenditure financing of the household, irrespective of any religious group. It means that both religious group, Hindus and Muslims are falling back upon borrowings to finance their health needs. In terms of affordability of healthcare services for social group the situation is very bad for SCs relative to their general counterpart all over the state. It is this group which is mostly falling back upon borrowings to finance their health expenditure. Their situation is particularly worst in Bundelkhand with wide gap of -7.76 between SC and general castes group. However, it is nearly close to five per cent in western and a bit lower in central and eastern regions in terms of borrowing as a source of financing of health consumption.

Now what is particularly important is the relative burden of treatment which is the lowest in western region. Central, eastern and Bundelkhand are having almost equal burden of treatment. However, this measure varies widely across socio-economic group among the four regions. It is rural, poor and marginalised section of society who is the worst suffers in terms of burden of treatment regardless of the region he/she may belong to. One can observe large variation in inequality on the basis of socio-economic characteristics among these four regions. It is the highest in Bundelkhand region followed by eastern UP and central UP. In UP nearly 20 per cent of the population does not seek formal care due to the lack of awareness; they didn't consider their diseases to be serious enough or took some tablets on casual suggestions or from medical shops. This shows the exclusion of certain group from the ambit of healthcare providers to consume healthcare. Most importantly a larger percentage doesn't go to the government health providers to seek care, only close to sixteen per cent availed the health facility from any public health institution.

Interestingly, percentage of persons seeking care on medical advice is the highest in western UP, nearly 87.6 per cent are seeking care on medical advice well above the states average, but their proportion in seeking care from government health facility is the lowest among the four regions of the state. As opposed to this in Bundelkhand and eastern region, lower percentage of people are seeking care on medical advice, but a larger percentage is seeking care from public health facility. In terms of socio-economic differential Muslims are worse off relative to Hindus in seeking formal healthcare. Again in terms of caste category lower caste people are more dependent on public healthcare services. As against this the people from general caste are more reluctant to seek care from public health providers, generally seeking care from high cost private health providers as nearly 95 per cent of people from the better off group reported taking healthcare on medical advice in all regions. Thus, it is mainly marginalised and poor who are going to public providers to seek treatment. Inequality among social group for seeking healthcare on medical advice is the highest in Bundelkhand and eastern region with wide gap of 7.71 and 6.48 respectively. Similar kind of pattern can be seen among Hindus and Muslims, rich and poor and rural and urban residence.

The malfunctioning of public health provisioning in backward regions of the state is clear from the fact that the number of OPD patient (male as well as female) in CHC is the highest in western region reflecting greater utilisation and acceptance of health services as against to this it is the lowest in eastern region followed by Bundelkhand. The utilisation of public health services for referral care is subsequently high in western UP even well above the states average. In western UP hospitalisation rate is just double of eastern UP. That means a larger section of poor is not going to seek referral care (hospitalisation treatment) in eastern UP. However, Eastern UP.

is having higher CMR that means high incidence of ailment and larger need for hospitalisation care. For the disease like diarrhea and acute respiratory tract infection the treatment taken from public health centres are on an average very low in UP with only 6.28 per cent children treated for diarrhea and only 7.99 per cent got treatment for acute respiratory tract infection. In regard to treatment of children for acute respiratory tract infection the utilisation is quite better in western UP (10.99), as opposed to Bundelkhand (2.92). In such a situation it can be easily guessed that those small percentages must be a section of population who are on higher or middle hierarchy of societal system and therefore poor and marginalised, yet not seeking care at all.

In order to have more explicit picture of public healthcare delivery it is important to look at availability, affordability and acceptability and utilisation of healthcare services in relation to health outcomes. But measuring health outcomes has various limitations of subjectivity where marginalised and poor may appear to enjoy better health outcomes due to the problem of underreporting and the element of subjectivity. Therefore, it can wrongly be inferred that they are enjoying better access to healthcare services too, which can't be the case as this is the section facing higher CMR which is taken as an objective indicator of health outcome.

However, inequality in health manifests itself into subjective and objective indicators. Inequalities based on subjective indicators are never captured fully, especially from indicators like morbidity (incidence of sickness). It tends to be higher for objective indicators of ill health like malnutrition and mortality. It is often noted that measures for the incidence of sickness sometimes produce wicked gradients with the better off reporting worse health than the poor whereas in reality this is not so.

The improved healthcare facilities and utilisation of public healthcare services are responsible for better health outcomes in any region. It can be shown that the reporting of ailment, Diarrhea and ARI among children is persistently high in western UP and it is consistently very low in eastern and Bundelkhand regions. Despite the fact that regions reporting lower morbidity are facing higher CMR as like western UP where it is having higher reporting of ailment with low level of CMR. It can be argued that inadequate and poorly equipped public health infrastructure jeopardizes access from several sides like poor quality of services at health centres, unavailability of health personnel etc. All this combined together result into bad health outcome along with increased inequality among the region. A very good example of such a case is eastern and Bundelkhand regions of UP where the underutilisation of public health services and worse health outcomes are persistent due to the underplay of public providers and they don't have purchasing power to attract private providers.

The inequality in Bundelkhand is exceptionally very high among religious group; it is 8.29 for acute ailment and 11.02 for chronic ailment. Similar kind of result can be seen for other ailment like diarrhea and fever among the children. If the poorer, rural and marginalised section of society is so prone to higher infant and child mortality, then the incidence of illness requiring hospitalisation may also be higher among them. Finally the high cost of treatment and hospitalisation may also act as a deterrent against seeking treatment, leading to prolongation of illness or even resulting into mortality in severe cases, apart from acting as a focus of infection in the community in the cases of infectious and communicable diseases.

A comparison of public health expenditure as percentage of GSDP of Kerala and UP from 1987-88 to 2007-08 reveals that it has been very low in UP from 1987. It has shown an improvement only after 2003-04 and from there onwards it is closer to Kerala's health expenditure. But earlier neglect of health sector in UP can't be compensated by the latter increase in public health expenditure. Moreover, that increase is too low to achieve the health goals. The real per capita public expenditure on health in Uttar Pradesh is far below the real per capita public health expenditure of Kerala. That means a small increase in absolute expenditure has been offset by the increased population and could not make any effective impact.

In UP the budgetary allocations on FW increased substantially in sup-periods while the dramatic decline in per capita spending on

Medical and PH reflects lack of life saving medical equipment and drugs in the health institutions. The programmes of Family Welfare have become the policy priority at national level. In the first five year plan it has been allocated about 3.3 per cent of national plan expenditures as part of World Bank project for population control. Particularly it has been more forcefully implemented in UP as it is the highest populous state facing highest growth rate of population. The altogether lower allocation of funding to health sector created low funding to general medicine and preventive care and as a result negligence of these sector. A study (Duggal, 2006) reveals a very alarming fact that in 1990s there have been improvements in primary health centres but the mobilisation of resources for FW converted these centres as machinery for population control and thereby missing their primary priority of ensuring primary healthcare services to all.

In subsequent years, at national level public investment strategy gave greater priority to economic growth and industrialisation with resultant reductions in health spending as a proportion of the total. During this period states health expenditure also decreased due to shrinkage of funding from centre. As a consequence of the fifth pay commission implementation around 1996-98 there has been shrinkage in non-salary components in the public health expenditure (Duggal, 2005). Thus, a greater reliance on the market for healthcare needs makes the access to healthcare services becomes more difficult for increasing number of poor in the state.

The evidence of galloping out of pocket expenditure and indebtedness for supporting healthcare expenditure is reflected from NSS 42nd and 52nd rounds and 60th round, where utilisation of health services has substantially increased and is being funded by the borrowings of the family. The major share of the resources has gone to curative services. As of 1990-91, a little more than 60 per cent of the resources have gone to curative services, 26 per cent to preventive services and the remaining into administration and miscellaneous services. This reflects a misallocation of resources in Uttar Pradesh, despite moderate increase in health expenditure in Uttar Pradesh. Further the average share of rural areas in healthcare expenditure is very low (33 per cent) in comparison to urban areas (66 per cent). Thus, the relationship between share of resources devoted to rural health sector and the share of rural population may not be in line with objective of achieving health for all (Bansal, 1999). Moreover, the public curative and hospital services are mostly in cities while in rural areas there are only preventive and promotive services like FP and immunisation. As a result private sector plays a very important role in health delivery system of rural areas especially in form of under-qualified medical professionals and quacks (Duggal, 2006).

In all indicators of mortality urban UP is better than rural UP. Interestingly, probability of survival of Muslim child is always better than Hindu child. All mortality rates are always higher in rural area and Hindu religious group. A child of a SC mother has lower chance of survival than any other caste groups. Wealth appears to improve child survival chances across all mortality rates. Therefore, it is the poor and marginalised facing highest mortality rate. Obviously these groups must be facing highest burden of ailment and as result are in a greater need of accessing public healthcare facilities at affordable price. In fact it is this group who are facing highest burden of disease in all regions of UP. Further, it is the poor and marginalised group of the society who are going to seek treatment from public providers for their health needs.

Over the year the decreasing expenditure and neglecting health policies have resulted into severe shortfall in health infrastructure as well health personnel in the state. As a result it has generated a smaller role for public providers. Consequently, the poor and people from lower strata of society are the worst affected by such compression in public health expenditure. Because the rich and better off section of the society can go to private providers due to their higher purchasing power, better negotiation capacity and social networks.

Thus, it is clear from above discussion that poor and marginalised people are the most likely to be ill and they are largely relying on public providers for their health needs. Therefore, it is this section which is worst affected by the shrinking of public healthcare expenditure and there by shrinking government role in provisioning of healthcare needs of the population. In fact there is already a very clear case of this section, largely dying in silence with a combination of highest mortality rate and lowest reporting of diseases. Therefore, if government further reduces its role in health sector, it is bound to affect health of the poor and marginalised.

Policy Implications and Suggestions

It needs to be emphasised that health is a peculiar kind of goods which is intrinsically as well as instrumentally important. Nature of demand for health is bound to be shaped by geographical location and individual characteristics. Therefore, supply of health needs to address specificities of demand also. In other words, health policy should be always unique for specific region and specific person. One universal health system or policy can't serve the need on equitable basis. Therefore for health sector a region specific need based policy is particularly required. This is all the more important in case of a heterogenous state like UP. The diversity of Uttar Pradesh definitely calls for a regions specific policy for its four regions. These regions vary drastically in terms of disease pattern, health outcomes, population and the socio-economic development. Health demand is not only determined by affordability only, rather it is more linked to social and cultural acceptance of health services and awareness about health needs. That is why health policy must have a regional orientation, especially in case of a state like Uttar Pradesh. Of course, recent initiatives like NRHM and URHM are an attempt to address region specific needs, but its result are yet to be realised.

It is the poor, SCs and Muslims who are found to be the worst in terms of proneness to diseases, burden of treatment and access to healthcare services. It is due to their low purchasing power, high cost of health services and unorganised and exploitative private sector. Therefore, it is particularly important for them to have affordable healthcare facilities that can be achieved either through reducing the cost of health facilities and drugs or providing some external support via insurance or cost coverage or discount at health institutions. This can be done by suitable targeting policies aimed at these groups. Moreover, only the existence of physical infrastructure is not sufficient for inclusive health system rather it should be accompanied by health personnel, necessary equipment and life saving drugs at affordable cost and at the approachable distance.

It is worth mentioning that Uttar Pradesh is characterised by high mortality and low morbidity. This is a unique situation which makes policy-making all the more complicated, which makes it difficult to gather information regarding the disease pattern in the state. A conscious examination and re-examination is required to formulate health policies. Therefore a stronger public health system is also required as a watch dog for the better monitoring of health status in the state.

It is not the absolute amount of public health expenditure only which matters in determining health outcomes. Rather, it is the composition of expenditure which has critically affected health outcomes and access to health in UP. This faulty composition has resulted into smaller and insignificant role for public providers in the health sector, promotion of urban and curative centric health policy and more attention on schemes of family planning at the cost of general health and medicine. Another important element which has resulted into underutilisation of public health resources is the mismatch between capital and revenue expenditure. Increased amount on capital expenditure with unmatched revenue expenditure has generated a scenario where hospital buildings are there but no health personnel, drugs etc is present there. Therefore, such policies, programmes and funds are required which can match and coordinate with each other.

In situation of macro-economic shocks the worst sufferers are poor and marginalised section of society since it is largely the poor and marginalised section of society which avails the public health facilities. Therefore in such a situation the policy of Public-Private-Partnership (PPP) is a good initiative but it needs to be suitably tailored by the government to safeguard the interest of downtrodden.

Inequality in health is generated by the combined operation of socio-economic characteristic and geographical location. That is why western UP faces the least inequality, whereas it is the highest in Bundelkhand, and SCs and other marginalised sections of former have better outcomes than same section of latter. Thus, social and economic development of a region has important bearings on access. Moreover the proactive state contributes extensively in reduction of health inequality as is evident from the health sector of Kerala. It has attained a more equitable and fair level of health outcomes despite its low level of economic growth. Similarly, better provisioning of health centres along with availability of health personnel reduced the health inequality in western UP. This is not possible in a region which has very small resources to share.

Work Cited

Bansal RD (1999): "Health Financing in India: Priorities, Issues, Inter- State Variations and Challenges", *Health and Population- Perspectives and Issues* 22 (3&4): 123-132.

Baru Rama, Acharya Arnab, Acharya Sanghmitra, Shiva AK, Nagraj K (2010): "Inequalities in access to Health Services in India: Caste, Class and Religion", *Economic and Political Weekly,* September 18, 2010, Vol. XLV No. 38.

Duggal Ravi (2006): "Utilisation of Health Care Services in India" in Prasad Sujata and Sathyamala C, *Securing Health For All: Dimensions and Challenges,* Institute for Human Development, New Delhi.

Gilson, Lucy and Schneider, Helen (2007): "Understanding Health Service Access: Concepts and Experience" in Stephen Matlin (Ed.) *Equitable Access: Research Challenge for Health in Developing Countries,* Global Forum Update on Research for Health Volume 4.

IIPS Macro International (2007): "National Family Health Survey" NFHS- 3, IIPS. Mumbai.

Meeta and Rajivlochan (2010): "Inequalities in Health, agrarian Distress and a Policy of Avoidance" *Economic and Political Weekly,* October 23, 2010, Vol. XLV No. 43.

Srivastava S Ravi (2006): "Health Security in Uttar Pradesh", in Prasad Sujata and Sathyamala C, *Securing Health For All: Dimensions and Challenges,* Institute for Human Development, New Delhi.

Simon T.D (2008): "Health Care Accessibility in Kerala: An Analysis across Different Socio-Economic Groups" Paper accepted for presentation at the Annual Conference on "*Equality, Inclusion and Human Development*" of the Human Development and Capability Association (HDCA), New Delhi, 10-13 September 2008.

State Planning Department (2007): "Human Development Report 2007" Government of Uttar Pradesh, Lucknow.

US Congress (1988): "*The Quality of Medical Care*", Office of the Technology Assessment, Publication No. OTAH – 386, US Government Printing Office, Washington DC.

Bibliography

Alkire S (2002): *Valuing Freedoms Sen's Capability Approach and Poverty Reduction,* Oxford University Press, New Delhi.

Anand P (2004): Capabilities and Health, *www.capability.approach.com/pubs/539anand_capabilities_health_pdf./.*, accessed on 10- 2-2010.

Anand S and Ravallion M (1993): "Human Development in Poor Countries: On the Role of Private Incomes and Public Services", *Journal of Economic Perspectives,* 1 (3).

Banerjee, A, Deaton A and Duflo E (2004): "Wealth Health, and Health Services in Rural Rajasthan", *American Economic Review* 94, No. 2, pp. 326-330.

Bansal RD (1999): "Health Financing in India: Priorities, Issues, Inter- State Variations and Challenges", *Health and Population- Perspectives and Issues* 22 (3&4): 123-132.

Baru Rama, Acharya Arnab, Acharya Sanghmitra, Shiva AK, Nagraj K (2010): "Inequalities in access to Health Services in India: Caste, Class and Religion", *Economic and Political Weekly,* September 18, 2010, Vol. XLV, No. 38.

Berman P (1991): "Health Economics, Health Financing and the Health Needs of Poor Women and Children in India", *The Ford Foundation,* New Delhi.

Berman P, Ahuja R and Bhandari L (2010): "The Impoverishing Effect of Healthcare Payments in India: New Methodology and Findings", *Economic and Political Weekly,* April 17, 2010, Vol. XLV No. 16.

Berman, J (2001): "Turning Point Initiative", *Colorado Department of Public Health and Environment,* pp. 37, 40, 44.

Bhalotra S: "Spending to Save? State Health Expenditure and Infant Mortality in India", *Department of Economics and CMPO, University of Bristol.*

Bidani B and Ravallion M (1997): "Decomposing Social Indicators Using Distributional Data", *Journal of Econometrics,* 77: 125-139.

Bloom E. David, Associates P River and Fang K (2001): "Social technology and human health", Concept paper for the Human Development Report 2001, *Channeling technology for Human Development.*

Bokhari Farasat AS, Gai Y, Gottret P (2007): "Government Health Expenditures and Health Outcomes", *Journal of Health Economics*, 16: 257-273.

Bose, A (2008): "Indias Disturbing Health Card", *Journal of Health Economics*, Vol. XLII, No. 50, pp. 10-13.

Creese A (1990): "User Charges for Healthcare: A Review of Recent Experiences", WHO, SHS Paper No. 1, Geneva.

Culyer AJ, Wagstaff A. (1993): "Equity and Equality in Health Care", *Journal of Health Economics*, 12: 431-457.

Dasgupta Rajib and Bisht Ramila (2010): "The Missing Mission in Health", *Economic and Political Weekly*, February 6, 2010, Vol. XLV No. 6.

Deolalikar AB (1995): "Government Health Spending in Indonesia: Impact on Children in Different Economic Groups" in Walle D and Nead K, *Public Spending and the Poor: Theory and Evidence*, Johns Hopkins University Press: Baltimore.

Department of Medicine (2010): "Introduction and Basic Information", Medicine and Health Care, *Government of Uttar Pradesh, website- govup.ac.in*

Desai Sapna (2009): "Keeping the Health in Health Insurance", *Economic and Political Weekly*, September 19, 2009, Vol. XLIV No. 38.

Dilip T.R. (2002): "Understanding Levels of Morbidity and Hospitalisation in Kerala, India", *Bulletin of the World Health Organisation* 2002, 80 (9).

Division of Economics and Statistics (2008): *Statistical Diary of Uttar Pradesh*, State Planning Institute, Department of Planning, Lucknow.

——— (2009-10): *Arthik Sameeksha*, State Planning Institute, Department of Planning, Lucknow.

Donnell OO, Doorslaer V Eddy, Wagstaff A and Lindelow M (2008): *"Analyzing Health Equity Using Household Survey Data: A Guide to Techniques and Their Implementation"*, The World Bank Washington, DC.

Donnell, OHeivan Doorslaer, Ravi R, Aparna Smanathan, Charu C Garg, Piya Hanvoravongchai, Mohammed N Huq, Anup K Karan, Gabriel M Leung, Keith in & Chitpranee Vasavid (2005): "Explaining the Incidence of Catastrophic Expenditures on Healthcare: Comparative Evidence from Asia", EQUITAP working Paper-5, Erasmus University, Colombo, Rotterdam and IPS.

Dorslaer V Eddy and Donnell O, (2008): "Measurement and Explanation of Inequalities in Health and Health Care in Low Income Settings", *UNU, WIDER*, Discussion Paper No. 04.

Drez and Sen (1995): *India : Economic Development and Social Opportunity*, Oxford University Press, New Delhi.

Dreze, Jean (2004): "Health Check-up", *The Hindu*, 12 March 2004.

Duggal Ravi (2001): "Health Sector Financing in the Context of Womens Health" in Mukhopadhyay Swapna, *Women's Health, Public and Community Action*, Manohar Publication, New Delhi.

———— (2005): "Public Health Expenditures, Investment and Financing Under the Shadow of a Growing Private Sector", in Gangolli V Leena, Duggal R and Shukla Abhay, *Review of Health Care in India,* Center for Equity into Health and Allied Themes (CEHAT).

———— (2006): "Utilisation of Health Care Services in India" in Prasad Sujata and Sathyamala C, *Securing Health For All: Dimensions and Challenges,* Institute for Human Development, New Delhi.

Duvvury Nata (1999): "Gender Implications of New Economic Policies", in Rao Mohan, *Disinvesting in Health: The World Bank's Prescriptions for Health,* Sage Publications, New Delhi.

Economic Research Foundation (2006): "Government Health Expenditure in India: A Benchmark Study", *MacArthur Foundation*, India.

EPW (2010): "Doctors for Rural India: What of the Proposal to Create a Cadre of Doctors Exclusively for Rural India?" *Economic and Political Weekly*, February 20, 2010, Vol. XLV No. 8.

Filmer D, Pritchett L (1999): "The Impact of Public Spending on Health: Does Money Matter?" *Social Science and Medicine* 49, 1309-1323.

Garg Charu and Anup Karan (2009): "Reducing Out of Pocket Expenditures to Reduce Poverty: A Disaggregated analysis at Rural and Urban and state Level in India", *Health Policy and Planning*, 24: 116-28.

Gilson, Lucy and Schneider, Helen (2007): "Understanding Health Service Access: Concepts and Experience" in Stephen Matlin (Ed.) *Equitable Access: Research Challenge for Health in Developing Countries,* Global Forum Update on Research for Health, Volume 4.

Girish K (2009): "Introduction: Health Sector Reforms in India: Issues, Experiences and Trends", in K Girish, *Health Sector Reforms in India,* Manohar, Centre De Sciences Humanities.

Global Forum for Health Research (2004): Health Research for Policy Action and Practice, http://www.who.int/alliance-hpsr/resources.

Government of India (2005): "Health Statistics of India", Ministry of Health and Family Welfare, Government of India.

Government of Uttar Pradesh (2006): "Human Development Report of Uttar Pradesh".

———— (2010): *Profile of Uttar Pradesh,* Government of Uttar Pradesh, website- govup.ac.in

Gupta Amit Sen (2004): "Misplaced Initiatives in the Health Sector", *People's Democracy,* Vol. XXVIII, no. 52, December- 26.

Gupta D Monica, B R Desikchari, Rajendra Shukla, T V Somanathan, P Padmanaban and KK Datta (2010): "How Might Indias Public Health Systems be Strengthened? Lessons from Tamil Nadu", *Economic and Political Weekly*, March 6, 2010, Vol. XLV No. 10.

Gupta I (2009): "Potential Impact on Health and Economic Inequality from Cardiovascular Diseases and Diabetes in India: Evidence from the National Sample Survey", *Discussion Paper Series No. 136/2009.*

Gupta S, Verhoeven M and Tiongson E (1999): "Does Higher Government Spending Buy Better Results in Education and Health Care?" *Washington DC: International Monetary Fund,* Working Paper 99/21.

Gupta Sanjeev, Verhoeven Marijn and Tiongson R Erwin (2002): "Public Spending on Health Care and the Poor", *Health Economics*, 12: 685- 696.

IIPS and Macro International (2007): National and Family Health Survey-3, 2005-06: India: vl1. Mumbai, IIPS.

IIPS and WHO (2006): "World Health Survey, 2003- India", International Institute for Population Sciences (IIPS), Mumbai, World Health Organisation, Geneva, World Health Organisation- India- WR Office, New Delhi.

IIPS Macro International (2007): "National Family Health Survey" NFHS- 3, IIPS, Mumbai.

International Institute for Population Sciences (IIPS) and Macro International (2008): "National Family Health Survey (NFHS-3), India, 2005- 06." IIPS, Mumbai.

Jalan B (2004): "Health and Wealth", *Biblio,* March- April 2004.

Johansson, Sheila Ryan and Carl Mosk (1987): "Exposure, Resistance and Life Expectancy: Disease and Death During the Economic Development of Japan, 1900- 1960", *Population Studies,* 41(2): 207-35.

John Jacob T (2010): "Is India Ready for an Overhaul in Healthcare?" *Economic and Political Weekly,* May 15, 2010, Vol. XLV No. 20.

Krishna A (2004): "Escaping Poverty and Becoming poor: Who Gains, Who Losses, and Why?" *World Development,* 32:121-36.

Krishnan TN (1999): "Access to Health and the Burden of Treatment in India: An Interstate Comparison", in Mohan Rao (ed.) *Disinvesting in Health: The World Bank's Prescription for Health*, Sage Publications, New Delhi, India.

Lorgelly PK, Lorimer K, Fenwick E, and Briggs AH (2008,a): Outcome Measurement in Economic Evaluations and the Role of the Capabilities Approach: A Review of the Literature, Section of Public Health Policy, University of Glasgow

———— (2008,b): The Capability Approach: Developing an Instrument for Evaluating Public Health Interventions, Section of Public Health Policy, University of Glasgow.

MacArthur Foundation (2006): "Government Health Expenditure in India: A Benchmark Study", *Economic Research Foundation,* New Delhi.

Martin MC (2008): "Individual and Collective Resources and Health in Morocco", *UNU- World Institute for Development Economic Research,* Research Paper No. 2008/21.

Mayer (2004): *The Intergenerational Impact of Health on Economic Growth,* Global Forum for Health Research, Forum 8.

Meeta and Rajivlochan (2010): "Inequalities in Health, agrarian Distress and a Policy of Avoidance" *Economic and Political Weekly,* October 23, 2010, Vol. XLV No. 43.

Minhas BS (1991): "Educational Deprivation and its Role as a Spoiler of Access to Better Life in India", *Indian Statistical Institute,* Technical Report No. 9104, Kolkata.

Ministry of Health and Family Welfare (2005): "Report of the National Commission on Macroeconomics and Health", Government of India.

——— (2007- 08): "District Level Household and Facility Survey under Reproductive and Child Health Project (DLHS-3)", International Institute of Population Sciences, Mumbai.

Mooij, J and Dev M (2002): "Social Sector Priorities: An Analysis of Budgets and Expenditures in India in the 1990s", *Development Policy Review* 22, No. 1, pp. 97-120.

Mukherjee AN, Karmakar K. (2008): "Untreated Morbidity and Demand for Healthcare in India: An Analysis of National Sample Survey Data", *Economic and Political Weekly*, November, 15.

Mukhopadhyay Swapna (1997): "Introduction", in Mukhopadhyay Swapna, *Women's Health, Public and Community Action,* Manohar Publication, New Delhi.

Narayana D (2010): "Review of the Rashtriya Swasthya Bima Yojana", *Economic and Political Weekly,* July 17, 2010, Vol. XLV No. 29.

Nathan, Mishra and Reddy, (2008): "An Alternative Approach to Measure HDI", *IGIDR, Mumbai,* Working Paper, 4.

National Sample Survey Organisation Reports on Various Rounds.

NIPFP (2005): "Health Care Status in India", National Institute of Public Finance and Policy, New Delhi.

Peter H David, Garg Anu, Bloom Gery, Walker G Damian, Brieger R William and Rahman M Hafizpur (2008): "Poverty and Access to Health Care in Developing Countries", *New York Academy of Sciences,* 1136: 161-171.

Pickett, K. E. and M. Pearl (2001): Multilevel analyses of neighbourhood socioeconomic context and health outcomes: a critical review. *Journal of Epidemiology and Community Health*, 55: 111-22.

Planning Commission (2008): "Report of the Study Group for Preparation of a Roadmap for Rapid Economic Development of Uttar Pradesh" *Government of India,* New Delhi.

Prabhu K Seeta (2001): *Economic Reform and Social Sector Development: A Study of Two Indian States*, United Nations Development Programme, New Delhi, Sage Publications, New Delhi.

———— (1999): "Structural Adjustment and the Health Sector in India", in Mohan Rao, *Disinvesting in Health: The World Bank's Prescription for Health*, Sage Publications, New Delhi.

Quadeer Imrana (1999): "The World Development Report 1993: The Brave New World of Primary Health Care", in Mohan Rao, *Disinvesting in Health: The World Bank's Prescription for Health*, Sage Publication, New Delhi.

Rao Govind M and Choudgary Mita: "Inter State Equalisation of Health Expenditure in Indian Union", *National Institute of Public Finance and Policy*, New Delhi.

Rao Mohan (1997): "Indias Augean Stables: The Unfinished Health Agenda" in Mukhopadhyay Swapna, *Women's Health, Public and Community Action*, Manohar Publication, New Delhi.

Ruger (2006,b): "Toward a Theory of a Right to Health: Capability and Incomplete Theorized Agreements", *Yale Journal of Law and Humanities*, Vol. 18:273.

———— (2007): "Rethinking Equal Access: Agency, Quality, and Norms", *Global Public Health*, January, 2(1): 78-96.

———— (2006,a): "Health, Capability, and Justice: Toward a New Paradigm of Health Ethics", Policy and Law, *Cornell Journal of Law and Public Policy*, Vol. 15:2.

———— (2004): "Health and Social Justice", *Public Health*, Vol. 364.

Ruta D, Camfield L, Donaldson, C (2007): "Sen and the Art of Quality of Life Maintenance: Towards a General Theory of Quality of Life and its Causation", *The Journal of Socio - Economics*, 36, 397-423.

Selvaraj Sakthivel and Karan K Anup (2009): "Deepening Health Insecurity in India: Evidence From National Sample Surveys since 1980s" *Economic and Political Weekly*, October 3, 2009, Vol. XLIV No. 40.

Sen A (1985): *Commodities and Capabilities*, New York, Elsevier.

———— (2002): "Why Health Equity", *Health Econ.* 11: 659-666.

———— (2004): "Many Faces of Gender Inequality in Rethinking Society in 21st Century: A Critical Readings in Sociology" in Michelle Webber and Kate Benzanson, *Canadian Scholars' Press Inc, Toronto, Ontario.*

Shariff Abusaleh and Mondal K Subrata (2009): "User Fee in Public Health Care Institutions" Ed. K Girish (2009): "Health Sector Reforms in India", *Manohar, Centre De Sciences Humanities.*

Simon T.D (2008): "Health Care Accessibility in Kerala: An Analysis across Different Socio-Economic Groups" Paper accepted for presentation at the Annual Conference on "*Equality, Inclusion and Human Development*" of the Human Development and Capability Association (HDCA), New Delhi, 10-13 September 2008.

Singh K Ajit (2000): *Uttar Pradesh Development Report 2000*, New Royal Book Company, Lucknow.

Srivastava S Ravi (2006): "Health Security in Uttar Pradesh", in Prasad Sujata and Sathyamala C, *Securing Health For All: Dimensions and Challenges,* Institute for Human Development, New Delhi.

State Planning Department (2007): *Human Development Report 2007,* Government of Uttar Pradesh, Lucknow.

Thorat S (2007): Economic Exclusion and Poverty: Indian Experience of Remedies Against Exclusion, Draft Prepared for Policy Forum, Agriculture and Rural Development for Reducing Poverty and Hunger in Asia: In Pursuit of Inclusive and Sustainable Growth, IFPRI.

Unni J (2009): "Gender Deferential in Education: Exploring the Capabilities Approach", *Economic and Political Weekly,* Vol. XLIV No.9.

US Congress (1988): *The Quality of Medical Care,* Office of the Technology Assessment, Publication No. OTAH – 386, US Government Printing Office, Washington D C.

Van, Doorslaer E, O O Donnell and R P Rannan- Elaja (2006): "Effects of Payments for Healthcare on Poverty in 11 Countries in Asia: An Analysis of Household Survey Data", *The Lancet,* 368: 1357-64.

Wagstaff A (2004): "The Millennium Development Goals for Health: Rising to the Challenges" World Bank Washington DC.

———— (2002): "Intersectoral Synergies and the Health MDGs: Preliminary Cross- Country Findings, Corroboration and Policy Simulations".

Wagstaff A, Paci P, Joshi H (2001): "Causes of Inequality in Health: Who You Are? Where You Live? Or Who Your Parents Were", *Policy Research Working Paper, 2713, World Bank, Washington, DC.*

Wagstaff, A and E Van Doorslaer (2003): "Catastrophe and Impoverishment in Paying for Healthcare: With Application to Vietnam 1993- 98", *Health Economics,* 12 (11): 921-34.

Wilkinson R, Marmot M (Ed.) (2003): *"Social Determinants of Health",* IInd Edition, International Centre for Health and Society, WHO.

World Bank (1995): "Public Expenditure Management for Sustained and Equitable growth", *World Bank Report* No. 14680- PH, Washington.

———— (2001): Engendering Development- through Gender Equality in Rights, Resources, and Voice. A Policy Research Report. New York: Oxford University press. Cited in (IIPS & Macro International, 2007, *National and Family Health Survey-3, 2005-06: India:* vl,1. Mumbai, IIPS).

Xu K D evans, G Carrian and A M Aguilar- Rivera (2005): "Designing Health Financing System to Reduce Catastrophic Health Expenditure" Number 2, Technical Brief for Policy Makers, *World Health Organisation, Department of Health System Financing.*

Annexure - A

Data and Methodology:

This study is based purely on secondary data source, namely–

1. Financial Accounts of Uttar Pradesh and Kerala for Various Years.
2. National Sample Survey, 2004 - 60th round survey during January-June 2004 of morbidity and utilisation of health services. The findings is based on published report as well as computation from unit record data.
3. NFHS – 3, the findings is based on published report (Vol. 2) as well as computation from unit record data.
4. DLHS – 3, the findings is based on published report- Uttar Pradesh, as well as computation from unit record data.

The present study is based on health service utilisation and morbidity data collected by NSS from its 60th round survey during January-June 2004. The enquiry regarding morbidity was with reference to the 15 days preceding the date of survey. For the ease of the study we divided ailment into acute, chronic and undiagnosed diseases. An acute disease lasts for just a short time, but can begin rapidly and have intense symptoms. In contrast, a chronic disease is likely to develop over time instead of having a sudden onset. Acute diseases for instance are frequent colds, influenza and sore throat etc. Medical intervention may make an individual with a chronic disease more comfortable, but usually chronic disease can't be cured and are potentially life threatening, for instance heart disease, cancer, diabetes etc. The undiagnosed diseases are those where the diagnosis is yet to be done. The prevalence of any ailment or its morbidity was calculated as following–

$$\text{Morbidity} = \frac{\text{No. of Persons Reporting Ailment during 15 days prior to Survey}}{\text{Total No. of the People in the Survey}}$$

Since the sample size at regional level becomes too small in NSS data, we have taken data of Diarrhoea and fever from DLHS - 3, 2007-08 in order to cross-check the case of under-reporting of morbidity. Therefore to cross-examine the pattern of morbidity we have taken data on morbidity from DLHS 3.

The differences in morbidity levels by selected background characteristics, known to be closely related to the health status of the population, are examined through cross-tabulation. Ailments reported during the survey were classified as acute or chronic to examine the prevalence of these conditions in various subsections of the population.

We then used NFHS-3 (2006-07) data set to get the details of objective health indicators which includes all categories of child mortality. However, we cannot use other valuable data of morbidity, utilisation of healthcare services given in NFHS-3 as this data set cannot be reduced at the district or regional level among the state. Therefore, to gather the information on those specific issues we have to substitute data from NSS 60th round and DLHS-3. The NFHS-3 has to be used because DLHS-3 and NSS do not provide data on child mortality. However, NSS collects data on mortality rate but its analysis has the limitations of small sample size when further dividing data into various sub-groups given the scarcity of the event.

We have used data from Facility Survey 2007-08 to analyse the availability of healthcare services among various region of Uttar Pradesh. Further we have to substitute data from NSS in order to look at the pattern of utilisation of public healthcare services and the affordability of these services among various sub-groups of the population. Facility Survey has the limitations in the sense that it does not provide data on the utilisation of healthcare services and its affordability. Therefore, we have to substitute data from NSS 60th round.

In order to study the affordability of public health services we have calculated burden of treatment. The following formula has been used to calculate burden of treatment-

$$\text{Burden of Treatment} = \frac{\text{Average Health Expenditure of the Household}}{\text{Average Consumption Expenditure of the Household}}$$

We have to substitute data in the place of NFHS-3 as it cannot be disaggregated at the regional level within the state.

To study the public health budget of the state we carried out trend analysis of the data from Financial Accounts of Uttar Pradesh and Kerala for various years. We calculated the trend of public health expenditure as a ratio of GSDP of the State. To calculate the trend of real per capita health expenditure we have first deflated the public health expenditure using GSDP deflator and then divided it by the population the state for each year.

Annexure - B

Table 1: Incidence of Ailment and CMR

State/Region	*Acute Ailment*	*Chronic Ailment*	*Undiag-nosed*	*Children Suffered from Diar-rhoeal*	*Children Suffered from ARI1*	*Number of Children***	*CMR-2001*
Uttar Pradesh	**25.8**	**20.64**	**1.47**	**16.2**	**16.9**	**48,551**	**95.69**
Western	32.67	25.19	1.53	19.373	20.99	19109	90.69
Central	28.19	21.08	2	14.67	16.99	6340	95.9
Eastern	18.27	16.55	1.32	11.17	12.11	3865	104.57
Southern	25.53	17.87	0.52	12.65	11.71	19237	91.59

Acute Ailment includes-

Chronic Ailment includes-

Undiagnosed-

Source: Computed by Author from NSS 60th Round.

Note: Table based on women with youngest living children born since 01.01.2004.

** Unweighted cases.

1 Last two weeks prior to survey.

† Represents figures for children of currently married women aged 15-44 years.

Table 2: Socio-economic Variation in the Utilisation of Services within the Region

	Western			
	BCG	**Polio**	**DPT**	**Measles Injection**
Hindu	69.15	97.09	53.12	44.66
Muslim	56.1	96.11	42.67	34.28
Caste				
Scheduled caste	68.48	96.99	53.44	42.84
Other backward class	62.51	96.55	47.46	39.04
Others	69.21	97.26	53.70	47.37
Sector				
Rural	65.94	96.65	49.95	41.09

Urban	62.57	97.49	50.66	44.05
Total	**65.27**	**96.81**	**50.09**	41.68

Central

	BCG	Polio	DPT	Measles Injection
Hindu	71.76	97.96	64	50.68
Muslim	58.33	97.47	49.02	35.78
Caste				
Scheduled caste	71.33	96.42	62.01	48.03
Other backward class	64.51	98.52	57.12	43.99
Others	77.66	97.87	69.15	57.98
Sector				
Rural	67.21	97.9	59.01	45.15
Urban	79.87	99.33	72.48	62.42
Total	**69.06**	**97.83**	**60.99**	**47.68**

Eastern

	BCG	Polio	BPT	Measles Injection
Hindu	71.25	98.16	66.02	51.52
Muslim	56.85	98.66	48.81	36.46
Caste				
Scheduled caste	68.01	97.8	60.56	44.81
Other backward class	66.75	98.39	61.88	47.03
Others	77.48	98.47	70.99	62.79
Sector				
Rural	68.86	98.24	63.04	48.49
Urban	63.7	98.52	58.52	50
Total	**68.46**	**98.26**	**62.68**	**48.61**

Southern

	BCG	Polio	DPT	Measles Injection
Hindu	78.46	96.95	66.56	54.66
Muslim	74	94	58	52
Caste				
Scheduled caste	82.68	94.97	73.18	56.98
Other backward class	75.84	97.47	61.8	51.97
Others	77.87	96.72	66.39	59.02
Sector				
Rural	76.79	96.34	63.7	53.23
Urban	86	99	79	62
Total	**78.16**	**96.73**	**65.97**	**54.53**

Table 3: Utilisation of Services in UP and its Regions

Region	*Any ANC*	*full2 Antenantal Checkup*	*BCG*	*DPT3*	*Polio*	*Measles*	*Percentage Received at least 1 dose of Vitamin A2*	*Number of Children*
Uttar Pradesh (15-49)	64.3	3.3	73.3	38.8	40.2	46.9	33.3	12,141
Western Region	58.68	2.90	72.92	35.63	37.98	45.55	32.38	4833
Central Region	59.41	3.83	74.98	41.01	41.61	49.94	36.89	1599
Bundelkhand Region	62.94	3.06	82.4	37.94	39.89	52.07	36.7	983
Eastern Region	75.87	4.28	75.52	46.26	46.68	49.92	35.25	4726

2 At least three visits for antenatal check-up, at least one TT injection received and 100+ IFA tablets/ syrup consumed.

Table 4. Socio-economic Variation in the Utilisation of Services within the Region

	Western	*Central*	*Eastern*	*Southern*	*Western*	*Central*	*Eastern*	*Southern*	*Western*	*Central*	*Eastern*	*Southern*
Religion	BCG	BCG	BCG	BCG	Polio	Polio	Polio	Polio	Measles Injection	Measles Injection	Measles Injection	Measles Injection
Religion												
Hindu	69.15	71.76	71.25	78.46	97.09	97.96	98.16	96.95	44.66	50.68	51.52	54.66
Muslim	56.1	58.33	56.85	74	96.11	97.47	98.66	94	34.28	35.78	36.46	52
Differential	**13.05**	**13.43**	**14.4**	**4.46**	**0.98**	**0.49**	**-0.5**	**2.95**	**10.38**	**14.9**	**15.06**	**2.66**
Caste												
Scheduled caste	68.48	71.33	68.01	82.68	96.99	96.42	97.8	94.97	42.84	48.03	44.81	56.98
Others	69.21	77.66	77.48	77.87	97.26	97.87	98.47	96.72	47.37	57.98	62.79	59.02
Differential	**-0.73**	**-6.33**	**-9.47**	**4.81**	**-0.27**	**-1.45**	**-0.67**	**-1.75**	**-4.53**	**-9.95**	**-17.98**	**-2.04**
Sector												
Rural	65.94	67.21	68.86	76.79	96.65	97.9	98.24	96.34	41.09	45.15	48.49	53.23
Urban	62.57	79.87	63.7	86	97.49	99.33	98.52	99	44.05	62.42	50	62
Differential	**3.37**	**-12.66**	**5.16**	**-9.21**	**-0.84**	**-1.43**	**-0.28**	**-2.66**	**-2.96**	**-17.27**	**-1.51**	**-8.77**

Table 5: Sources of Treatment in Regions by Characteristics

Source of Treatment	*Treatment Taken on Medical Advice*				*Utilisation of Government Hospitals*			
Region	*Western*	*Central*	*Eastern*	*Southern*	*Western*	*Central*	*Eastern*	*Southern*
	87.6	77.18	76.82	76.19	11.86	21.56	16.01	26.34
Religion								
Hindu	97.22	93.81	95.46	92.29	11.13	23.63	17.62	25.89
Muslim	93.58	93.64	88.98	100	12	7.89	10.23	30.48
Caste								
Scheduled caste	98.06	93.37	98.27	90.09	12.18	29.93	20.11	30.77
OBC	96.18	94	95.33	92.11	11.38	13.97	13.38	20.97
Others	95.65	93.74	89.3	97.44	10.71	22.74	19.37	30.49
Sector								
Rural	87.42	70.36	75.39	60.73	10.14	20.42	15	31.51
Urban	88.02	90.4	83.09	77.3	15.58	24.27	13.36	22.31
MPCE-Class								
0- 300	85.32	67.71	70.24	64.52	18.39	23.73	17.71	30
300- 600	88.24	72.84	75.84	60.25	9.42	20.09	14.18	30.94
600- 900	85.31	81.01	85.2	77.45	14.22	22.4	12.57	22.67
900 & above	90.04	91.62	82.73	86.84	14.89	24.48	16.36	21.21

Table 6: Source of Informal Treatment

	No Formal Treatment											
	Self/Other/HH/Friend				*Medical Shop*				*Other*			
Region	*Western*	*Central*	*Eastern*	*Southern*	*Western*	*Central*	*Eastern*	*Southern*	*Western*	*Central*	*Eastern*	*Southern*
	13.75	14.84	15.28	18.32	25.75	39.78	43.52	30.69	59.75	45.38	41.2	50.99
Religion												
Hindu	24.18	5	22.06	11.76	23.08	31.25	61.76	41.18	52.75	63.54	16.18	47.06
Muslim	1	0	0	0	60.76	7.41	37.25	0	37.97	92.59	62.75	0
Caste												
Scheduled caste	22	0	0	60	44.44	41.94	0	10	33.33	58.06	100	30
OBC	6.42	10.42	26.92	0	44.04	20.83	71.15	52.94	49.54	68.75	1.92	47.06
Others	27.91	0	1.64	0	30.23	20.45	39.34	28.57	41.86	79.55	59.02	71.43
Rural	19.01	15.71	18.13	11.11	15.49	31.41	36.81	18.52	64.79	52.88	45.05	70.37
Urban	7.94	0	27.78	13.04	58.73	95.24	61.11	39.13	33.33	4.76	11.11	47.83
MPCE-Class												
0- 300	20	15.91	9.62	40	0	40.91	34.62	40	80	43.18	55.77	20
300- 600	12.71	15.08	21.31	7.55	19.49	33.33	44.26	24.53	66.95	51.59	34.43	67.92
600- 900	20.9	8.82	23.81	16.67	44.78	44.12	19.05	22.22	34.33	47.06	57.14	61.11
900 & above	13.33	12.5	40	0	40	62.5	40	0	46.67	25	20	100

Western	*Average Expenditure*	*Expenses Borrowings*	*Expenses Contribution*	*Expenses Other Sources*
Religion				
Hindu	633.88	8.89	1.26	0.89
Muslim	475.13	5.47	1.83	2.10
Caste				
Scheduled caste	614.97	11.21	1.83	0.82
Other backward class	545.33	8.39	1.15	1.56
Others	674.51	5.66	1.06	0.72
Central				
Religion				
Hindu	587.25	4.48	3.37	2.60
Muslim	596.45	5.39	5.02	2.45
Caste				
Scheduled caste	456.51	7.46	5.09	2.96
Other backward class	459.16	4.54	2.91	1.57
Others	827.76	3.13	3.84	3.56

(Contd...)

Eastern				
Religion				
Hindu	688.77	6.24	1.51	2.37
Muslim	505.01	3.62	1.97	1.18
Caste				
Scheduled caste	595.64	8.97	1.81	2.22
Other backward class	690.26	5.19	2.08	2.10
Others	616.23	4.55	0.52	2.13
Southern				
Religion				
Hindu	573.08	8.47	2.92	0
Muslim	403.67	11.43	0	0
Caste				
Scheduled caste	503.98	17.34	3.72	0
Other backward class	433.71	3.01	1.69	0
Others	824.46	9.58	3.19	0

Table 7: Distribution of Expenditure by Source of Finance

	Average Total Expenditure	*Household Income/ Saving*	*Expenses Borrowings*	*Percentage Borrowed*	*Expenses Contribution*	*Percentage Get Contribution*	*Expenses Other Sources (other sources (incl. sale of ornaments and other physical assets, draught animals, etc.)*	*Percentage-Other Sources*
Western	**637.79**	**596.66**	**1112.85**	**8.09**	**730.16**	**1.25**	**430.69**	**1.17**
Religion								
Hindu	671.849	633.88	1086.65	8.89	797.51	1.26	359.23	0.26
Muslim	508.52	475.13	1251.81	5.47	496.66	1.19	477.3	0.40
Social Group								
Scheduled caste	590.14	614.97	744.72	11.21	530.77	1.83	889.68	0.82
Other backward class	583.94	545.33	1179.84	8.39	316.62	1.15	424.97	1.56
Others	748.6	674.51	1385.57	5.66	1719.7	1.06	133.04	0.72
Sector								
Rural	616.69	607.71	1050.67	9.44	445.44	1.55	483.27	1.30
Urban	676.24	574.62	1329.53	5.40	2104.26	0.64	282.51	0.92
MPCE-Class								
0- 300	406.86	417.52	770.6	13.48	543.75	2.91	505.33	0.55
300- 600	509.83	516.24	940.15	9.28	348.61	1.51	248.6	0.33
600- 900	585.7	603.35	1080.47	5.88	763.62	0.56	246.5	0.21
900 & above	1149.45	1019.2	2959.85	5.16	4109.09	0.82	2175	0.15

Table 8: Distribution of Expenditure by Source of Finance

	Average Total Expenditure	*Household Income/ Saving*	*Expenses Borrow-ings*	*Percentage Borrowed*	*Expenses Contri-bution*	*Percentage Get Contri-bution*	*Expenses Other Sources*	*Percentage Other Sources*
Central	594.05	589.14	2081.01	4.66	525.51	3.71	874.31	2.57
Religion								
Hindu	584.07	587.25	2276.77	4.48	372.51	3.37	867.56	0.73
Muslim	641.69	596.45	1453.68	5.39	921.04	5.02	509.11	1.10
Social Group								
Scheduled caste	466.83	456.51	608.01	7.46	444.88	5.09	946.04	2.96
Other backward class	480.32	459.16	1802.74	4.54	490.96	2.91	934.59	1.57
Others	786.45	827.76	4683.36	3.13	621.7	3.84	805.9	3.56
Sector								
Rural	598.99	598.99	1554.03	8.39	380.22	5.89	940.76	2.50
Urban	583.43	583.43	854.72	3.48	550.9	6.96	569.53	4.75
MPCE-Class								
0- 300	420.95	420.95	659.16	9.45	405	3.94	801.62	6.30
300- 600	554.86	554.86	1828	8.03	388.52	3.82	783.63	2.21
600- 900	651.81	651.81	613.46	6.82	458.17	13.18	859.72	5.00
900 & above	786	786	7750	0.67	515	6.00	23	1.33
Eastern	597.15	652.46	1555.58	5.72	498.2	1.60	642.04	2.13
Religion								
Hindu	614.8	688.77	1678.89	6.24	368.84	1.51	745.75	0.56
Muslim	532.2	505.01	692.39	3.62	901.8	1.97	816.66	0.24
Social Group								
Scheduled caste	589.48	595.64	1099.35	8.97	501.13	1.81	998.22	2.22
Other backward class	587.1	690.26	2231.57	5.19	520.55	2.08	592.53	2.10
Others	622.32	616.23	644.81	4.55	312.22	0.52	479.81	2.13
Sector								
Rural	610.39	610.39	994.4	7.11	503.66	2.13	746.27	2.95
Urban	544.63	544.63	1304	4.03	378.5	4.03	811.66	1.21
MPCE-Class								
0- 300	388.23	388.23	518.75	5.83	50	0.49	350	0.97
300- 600	538.85	538.85	1080.53	6.00	612.95	3.07	734.8	2.93
600- 900	845.5	845.5	571	7.69	137.5	1.03	1101.33	3.08
900 & above	916.61	916.61	2139.5	8.77	92	5.26	446	2.63
Total		**609.36**	**1319.98**	**6.83**	**596.25**	**1.86**	**633.99**	**1.64**

Southern	**564.66**	**557.85**	**856.47**	**8.73**	**678.7**	**2.65**	**0**	**0.00**
Religion								
Hindu	573.51	573.08	886.56	8.47	678.7	2.92	0	0.00
Muslim	444.1	403.67	630.75	11.43	0	0.00	0	0.00
Social Group								
Scheduled caste	606.4	503.98	471.94	17.34	826.25	3.72	0	0.00
Other backward class	423.21	433.71	1159.12	3.01	391.66	1.69	0	0.00
others	731.26	824.46	1412.83	9.58	760	3.19	0	0.00
Sector								
Rural	626.68	626.68	652.52	10.98	702.22	0.00	0	0.00
Urban	488.56	488.56	748.71	4.96	0	0.00	0	0.00
MPCE-Class								
0- 300	402.24	402.24	230	8.00	0	0.00	0	0.00
300- 600	508.45	508.45	692.45	11.76	489.375	4.71	0	0.00
600- 900	673.63	508.45	443.33	3.53	872.5	11.76	0	0.00
900 & above	692.73	692.73	2000	2.94	0	0.00	0	0.00
Total		**609.36**	**1319.98**	**6.83**	**596.25**	**1.86**	**633.99**	**1.64**

Table 9: Reason for No Treatment

	No medical available in the neighbour-hood	*Facilities available but no treatment sought owing to: lack of faith*	*Long waiting*	*Financial reasons*	*Ailment not considered serious*	*Others*
Region						
Western	20.45	5.52	0.32	26.62	37.34	9.74
Religion						
Hindu	20.89	6.22	0.44	27.11	34.67	10.67
Muslim	20	3.75	0	26.25	43.75	6.25
Caste						
Scheduled caste	21.13	1.41	0	38.03	33.8	5.63
Other backward class	21.05	7.24	0.66	23.68	37.5	9.87
Others	19.51	6.1	0	20.73	40.24	13.41
Sector						
Rural	29.17	6.48	0	25.46	31.48	7.41
Urban	0	3.26	1.09	29.35	51.09	15.22

MPCE-Class						
0- 300	23.08	7.69	0	7.69	53.85	7.69
300- 600	24.55	7.19	0	28.74	29.34	10.18
600- 900	14.42	2.88	0.96	30.77	43.27	7.69
900 & above	16.67	4.17	0	4.17	58.33	16.67
Central	24.16	2.6	1.12	32.71	27.51	11.9
Religion						
Hindu	28.32	3.1	0	28.32	27.43	12.83
Muslim	2.33	0	6.98	55.81	27.91	6.98
Caste						
Scheduled caste	31.58	2.63	0	28.95	25	11.84
Other backward class	16.22	3.6	0	36.94	31.53	11.71
Others	28.05	1.22	3.66	30.49	24.39	12.2
Sector						
Rural	26.97	2.9	1.24	31.12	25.73	12.03
Urban	0	0	0	46.43	42.86	10.71
MPCE-Class						
0- 300	12.73	0	0	47.27	32.73	7.27
300- 600	27.22	2.96	1.78	30.18	24.26	13.61
600- 900	32.43	0	0	27.03	29.73	10.81
900 & above	0	25	0	12.5	50	12.5
Eastern						
Religion						
Hindu	13.14	9.75	0.85	30.51	38.98	6.78
Muslim	5.77	17.31	0	30.77	32.69	13.46
Caste						
Scheduled caste	15.87	9.52	1.59	33.33	30.16	9.52
Other backward class	13.77	12.32	0	37.68	31.88	4.35
Others	5.81	9.3	1.16	17.44	53.49	12.79
Sector						
Rural	13.23	12.45	0.39	29.18	36.19	8.56
Urban	0	0	3.23	41.94	51.61	3.23
MPCE-Class						
0- 300	11.43	22.86	0	37.14	18.57	10
300- 600	12.29	8.38	1.12	26.82	44.13	7.26

600- 900	10.71	3.57	0	42.86	35.71	7.14
900 & above	9.09	0	0	18.18	63.64	9.09
Southern	3.91	1.56	0.78	40.63	39.84	13.28
Religion						
Hindu	4.13	1.65	0.83	41.32	38.84	13.22
Muslim	0	0	0	28.57	57.14	14.29
Caste						
Scheduled caste	3.45	3.45	0	55.17	17.24	20.69
Other backward class	3.9	0	1.3	37.66	44.16	12.99
Others	5	5	0	25	60	5
Sector						
Rural	5.49	2.2	0	40.66	38.46	13.19
Urban	0	0	2.7	40.54	43.24	13.51
MPCE-Class						
0- 300	0	10	0	30	30	30
300- 600	4.35	0	1.09	45.65	39.13	9.78
600- 900	4.35	0	0	26.09	52.17	17.39
900 & above	0	33.33	0	33.33	0	33.33

Table: 10- Burden of Diseases

	Western		Burden of Disease	Western		Burden of Disease	Western		Burden of Disease	Western		Burden of Disease
Sector	*Average Annual Per capita Expenditure of HH*	*Average Treatment Cost*		*Average Annual Per capita Expenditure of HH*	*Average Treatment Cost*		*Average Annual Per capita Expenditure of HH*	*Average Treatment Cost*		*Average Annual Per capita Expenditure of HH*	*Average Treatment Cost*	
Rural	3456.73	616.69	17.84	2646.07	598.99	22.64	2946.15	610.39	20.72	2876.08	626.68	21.79
Urban	4818.3	676.24	14.03	4304.65	583.43	13.55	4429.13	544.63	12.30	3289.58	488.56	14.85
Religion												
Hindu	3927.15	671.84	17.11	3134.52	584.07	18.63	3122.75	614.8	19.69	2993.06	573.51	19.16
Muslim	3912.35	508.52	13.00	3183.15	641.69	20.16	3607.42	532.2	14.75	3282.2	444.1	13.53
Social Group												
SC	3049.61	590.14	19.35	2277.14	466.83	20.50	2402.16	589.48	24.54	2527.34	606.4	23.99
OBC	3662.84	583.94	15.94	2949.67	480.32	16.28	3140.88	587.1	18.69	2854.19	423.21	14.83
General	4981.21	748.6	15.03	4032.85	786.45	19.50	3988.28	622.32	15.60	3977.18	731.26	18.39
MPCE Class												
0-300	2086.84	406.86	19.50	1683.12	420.95	25.01	1957.02	388.23	19.84	1707.71	402.24	23.55
300-600	3082.2	509.83	16.54	2608.74	554.86	21.27	2881.69	538.85	18.70	2680.06	508.45	18.97
600-900	4094.82	585.7	14.30	3408.3	651.81	19.12	3978.12	845.5	21.25	3592.08	673.63	18.75
900 & Above	6585.15	1149.45	17.46	6457.51	786	12.17	6850.77	916.61	13.38	4600.73	692.73	15.06
Total	**3949.57**	**637.79**	**16.15**	**3157.55**	**594.05**	**18.81**	**3198.97**	**597.15**	**18.67**	**3040.07**	**564.66**	**18.57**

Annexure - C

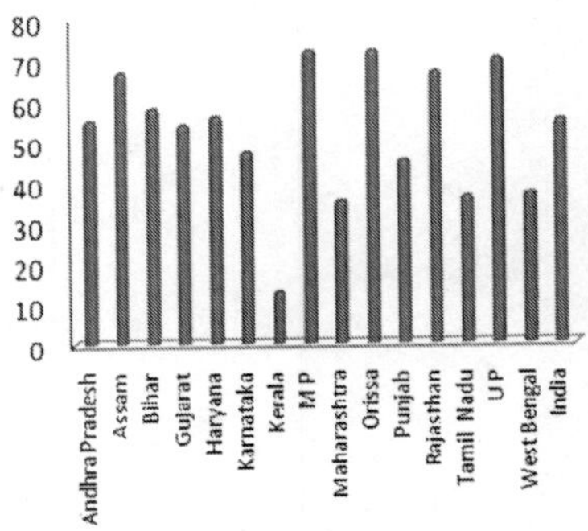

Figure 1a: Life Expectancy at Birth- 2002- 06.

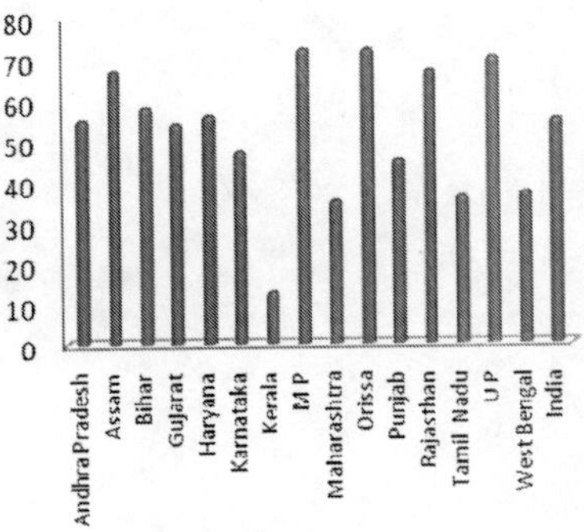

Figure 1b: Infant Mortality - 2007.

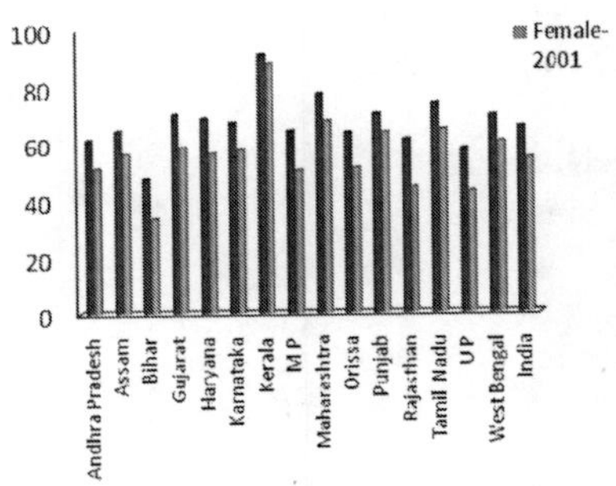

Figure 1c: Total Fertility Rate by State.

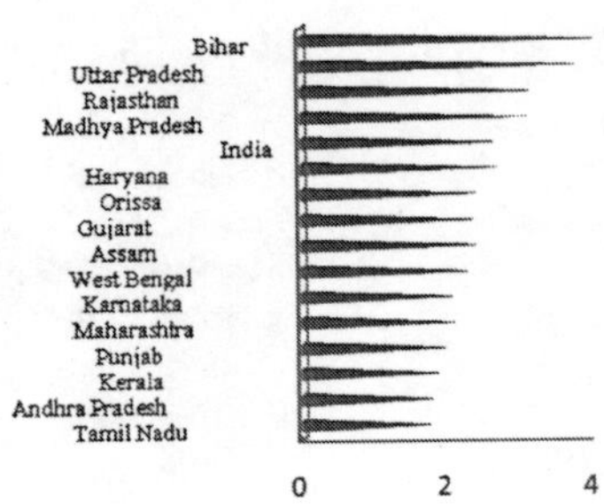

Figure 1d: Literacy Rate- 2001.

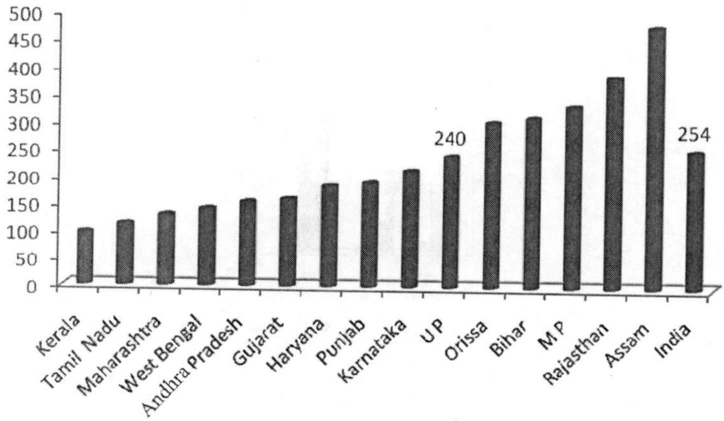

Figure 1e: Meternal Mortality-2004-05.

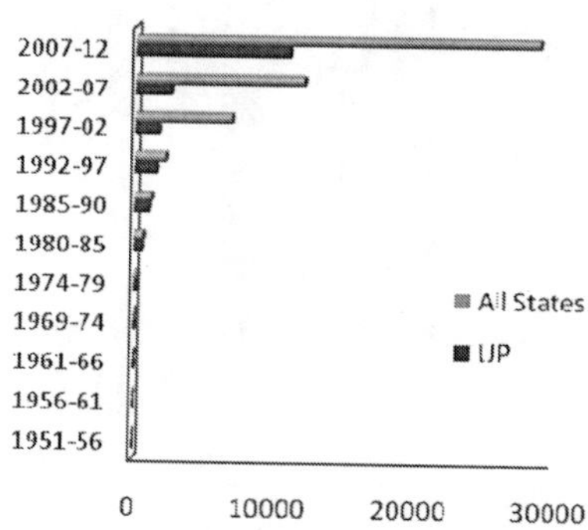

Figure 2a: Per Capita Plan Expenditure in UP and All States.

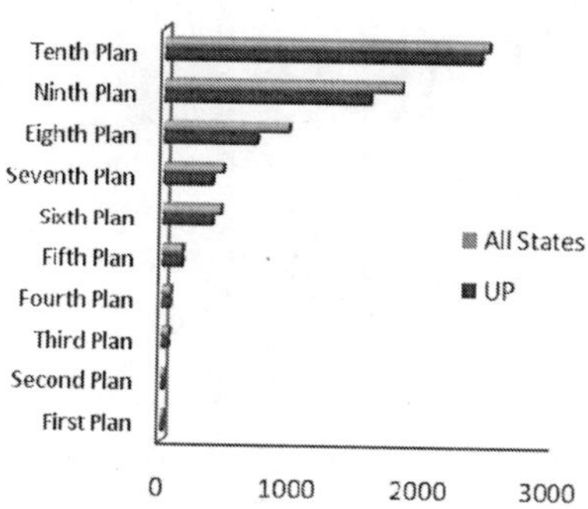

Figure 2b: Per Capita Plan Assistance in UP and All States.

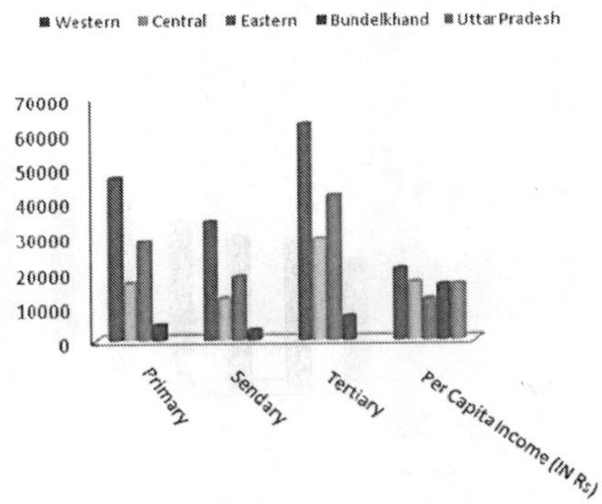

Figure 3a: NDDP By Economic Activity-2007-08.

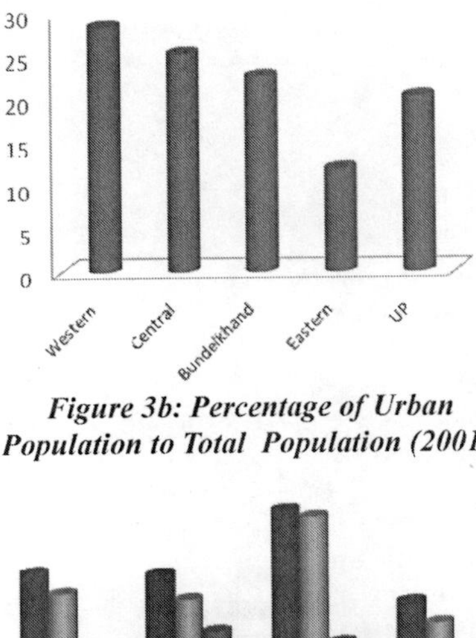

Figure 3b: Percentage of Urban Population to Total Population (2001).

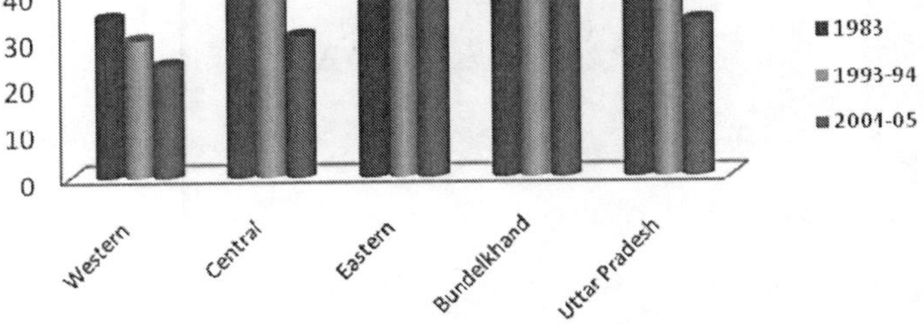

Figure 3c: Regional Incidence of Poverty in Rural UP.

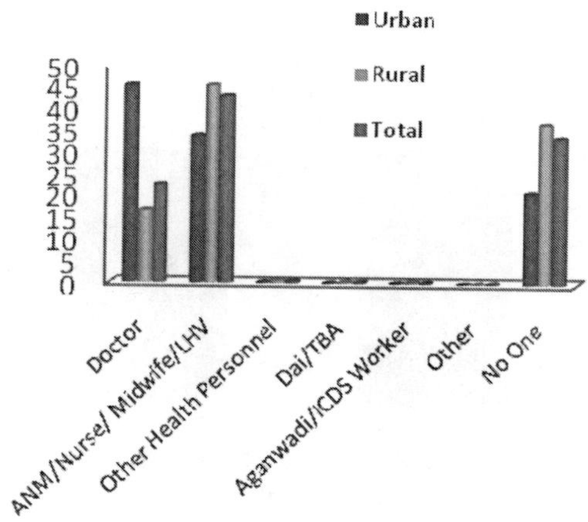

Figure 4a: ANC Provider During Pregnancy - 2006-07.

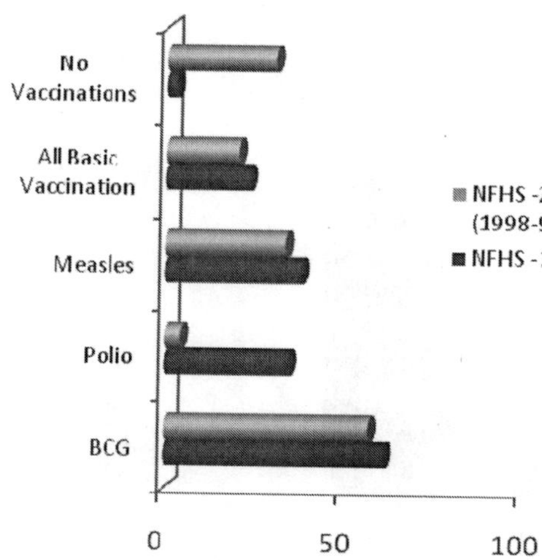

Figure 4b: Trend in Vaccination Coverage.

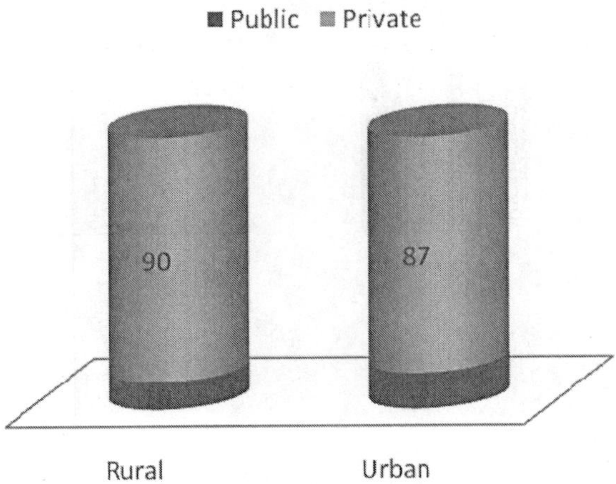

Figure 5a: Out-patient Services - UP.

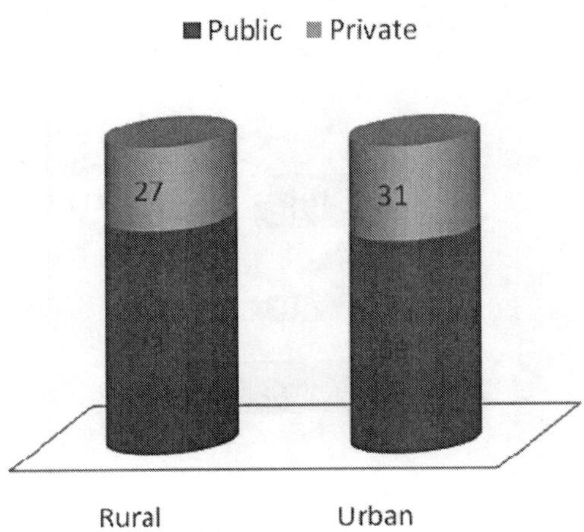

Figure 5b: Patient Services - UP.

Index

I

J & L

M

N

O

P